£19.99 ✓

Midwife's Guide to Antenatal Investigations

For Elsevier:

Commissioning Editor: Mary Seager
Development Editor: Rebecca Nelemans
Project Manager: Andrew Palfreyman
Designer: Andy Chapman
Illustration Buyer: Gillian Murray
Illustrator: Jane Fallows

Midwife's Guide to Antenatal Investigations

£19.99

Edited by

Amanda Sullivan BA(Hons) PGDip PhD RM RGN

Consultant Midwife, Nottingham University Hospital NHS Trust, Nottingham, UK

Lucy Kean BM BCH DM MRCOG

Consultant Obstetrician, Subspecialist in Fetal and Maternal Medicine, Nottingham University Hospitals NHS Trust, Nottingham, UK

and

Alison Cryer SRN SCM

Regional Coordinator Antenatal Screening Programmes, East Midlands, UK

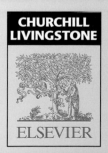

CHURCHILL LIVINGSTONE

ELSEVIER

Edinburgh London New York Oxford Philadelphia St Louis Sydney Toronto 2006

CHURCHILL
LIVINGSTONE
ELSEVIER

First Edition 2006

ISBN 10: 0 443 10141 8
ISBN 13: 978 0 443 10141 0

British Library Cataloguing in Publication Data
A catalogue record for this book is available from the British Library

Library of Congress Cataloging in Publication Data
A catalog record for this book is available from the Library of Congress

Knowledge and best practice in this field are constantly changing. As new research and experience broaden our knowledge, changes in practice, treatment and drug therapy may become necessary or appropriate. Readers are advised to check the most current information provided (i) on procedures featured or (ii) by the manufacturer of each product to be administered, to verify the recommended dose or formula, the method and duration of administration, and contraindications. It is the responsibility of the practitioner, relying on their own experience and knowledge of the patient, to make diagnoses, to determine dosages and the best treatment for each individual patient, and to take all appropriate safety precautions. To the fullest extent of the law, neither the publisher nor the editors assumes any liability for any injury and/or damage.

The Publisher

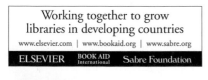

Working together to grow
libraries in developing countries

www.elsevier.com | www.bookaid.org | www.sabre.org

ELSEVIER   BOOK AID International   Sabre Foundation

ELSEVIER   your source for books,
journals and multimedia
in the health sciences

www.elsevierhealth.com

The
Publisher's
policy is to use
paper manufactured
from sustainable forests

Printed in China by CTPS

Contents

Contributors

Jane Fisher
Director, Antenatal Results and Choices (ARC), London, UK

Donna Holdcroft MPhil DCR(R) DMU DMS
Programme Leader MSc Medical Ultrasound, University of Derby, Derby, UK

Lucy Kean BM BCH DM MRCOG
Consultant Obstetrician and Subspecialist in Fetal and Maternal Medicine, Nottingham City Hospital, Nottingham, UK

Donna Kirwan RGN RM PGCertDU
Northwest Regional Coordinator, Antenatal Screening Programmes, Liverpool, UK

Ellen Knox MBChB MRCOG
Specialist Registrar Obstetrics and Gynaecology, Birmingham Women's Hospital, Birmingham, UK

Pam Loughna MD FRCOG MRCGP
Senior Lecturer and Consultant Obstetrician, Academic Division of Obstetrics and Gynaecology, Nottingham University Hospitals NHS Trust, Nottingham, UK

William Martin MRCOG DM
Consultant Fetal Maternal Medicine, Birmingham Women's Hospital, Birmingham, UK

Ann Minton M Med Ed BSC(Hons) DCR(R) DMU
University Principal Tutor, University of Derby, Derby, UK

Andrew Simm MB ChB MRCOG
Consultant Obstetrician with Special Interest in Feto-Maternal Medicine, Nottingham University Hospitals NHS Trust, Nottingham, UK

Jane Strong MBChB MRCP(UK) MRCPath
Consultant Haematologist, Leicester Royal Infirmary, Leicester, UK

Amanda Sullivan BA(Hons) PGDip PhD RM RGN
Midwife Consultant, Nottingham University Hospitals NHS Trust, Nottingham, UK

Carine Vassy PhD
Senior Lecturer in Sociology, University of Paris B, Bobigry, France

Pat Ward RN RM CHSM MA
National Programme Director, Down's Syndrome and Fetal Ultrasound Anomaly Screening, Northants, UK

Preface

Antenatal investigations are a vital part of antenatal care. They shape the way that care is delivered. Routine bookings involve at least nine tests. Additional procedures are instigated on a case-by-case basis. This book therefore brings together expertise from the relevant specialties, to provide an accessible guide for midwives. The book is designed for easy reference during a busy clinic or heavy clinical workload. It can also be used to educate students and update practising midwives. Emphasis is placed on how to communicate with women when offering tests and when giving the results. Normal parameters and findings that require follow-up are also identified. Case examples are given and each chapter highlights key practice points.

The first section puts antenatal investigations in context. Chapter 1 describes how certain investigations developed and became embedded into routine care. The impact on women's perceptions and experiences of pregnancy is also discussed. This background information is important in assisting clinicians to understand how technologies have evolved and why services are arranged as they are. The societal impact of testing may not be readily apparent to the midwife amidst the day-to-day pressures of delivering a clinical service.

Chapter 2 aims to equip midwives with the knowledge needed to communicate with parents and to help them through the testing process. Terminology that is commonly used to describe test performance is explained and sources of further information are highlighted. Chapter 3 focuses on pregnancy loss, breaking bad news and supporting parents. The chapter author is the Director of the charity Antenatal Results and Choices (ARC). This charity supports parents throughout antenatal testing and is an educational resource for professionals.

Sections 2 and 3 describe the application and interpretation of antenatal investigations in clinical practice. Section 2 is concerned with maternal investigations and is divided into key topic areas. The first of these is haematology in pregnancy (Ch. 4). This includes an explanation of normal haematological indices and normal pregnancy ranges. Screening and management of haemoglobinopathies are also explained in line with recent policy changes. The management of potential haemolytic disease of the newborn and maternal autoimmune antibodies are also explained. This chapter condenses complex haematology into a format that is accessible for midwives.

The next main topic is maternal disease in pregnancy (Ch. 5). This incorporates maternal disorders, such as diabetes and hypertension. The recognition and management of intrahepatic cholestasis of pregnancy is also made clear. The final topic in this section covers infections in pregnancy, such as hepatitis B, varicella and parvovirus. All topics were selected because they are regularly encountered in clinical practice, but can cause confusion.

Section 3 is concerned with fetal investigations. This section includes first and second trimester ultrasound scans (Chs. 7 and 8). Common ultrasound findings are explained using annotated images. These chapters demonstrate how ultrasound is applied to routine antenatal care and fetal structures that are examined. It is crucial that midwives understand this, so that they are equipped to discuss the procedure with parents. Chapter 9 describes how biochemical markers in maternal serum can be used to assess the risk of fetal anomaly. Serum biochemical markers for Down's syndrome are described, since new markers have been identified and added to the national screening programme.

Ultrasound findings and maternal serum biochemistry can lead to fetal chromosome or genetic testing. Accordingly, Chapter 10 describes common indications for testing and the aetiology of chromosomal abnormalities. Procedures such as chorionic villus sampling and amniocentesis are also explained. Midwives are often called upon to discuss the risks and benefits of these tests with parents. This section concludes by explaining when and how fetal wellbeing assessments should be performed. The place for biophysical profiling and Doppler measurement of fetal blood flow is also made clear.

The final section of the book considers how new and emerging technologies are likely to influence midwifery roles in the future. Technological developments have altered women's experiences of preg-nancy and will continue to do so. There will be new ethical dilemmas, particularly in the field of genetics. New midwifery roles are also discussed. To conclude, this book aims to help midwives comprehend and interpret the range of antenatal investigations that are used in everyday practice. It bridges the divide between complex specialist knowledge and basic texts. It is a handbook for all midwives involved in the delivery of antenatal care.

Amanda Sullivan
Lucy Kean
Alison Cryer

Section One

Clinical practice in context

SECTION CONTENTS

1

The development of fetal investigations: historical and sociological perspectives

Carine Vassy

CHAPTER CONTENTS

INTRODUCTION

Social sciences can help clinicians to deepen their understanding of the social and psychological effects of antenatal investigations, as these are often not apparent in the clinical area. This chapter presents a brief historical perspective on the development of fetal investigations and a sociological analysis of their impact. The focus on fetal investigation techniques is all the more important in that they have had the main effect on women's experience of pregnancy. The aim of this chapter is to explain how they became embedded within antenatal care and what new questions they have raised about the definition of normality and life.

Antenatal care dramatically changed in the twentieth century with great progress being made in improving the health of women and newborns. Some of the most well-known advances were fetal-investigation techniques. The main aims of these techniques are to confirm fetal viability, diagnose multiple pregnancies, check the localisation of the placenta to avoid problems for the delivery, and detect any congenital or constitutional abnormalities in fetal development.

The aim of detecting abnormality is the most controversial because the problem that has been identified can rarely be cured. Often the only available intervention is medical abortion. Therapeutic interventions are not as advanced as diagnostic tools. Fetal surgery is still at an experimental stage. Some observers adopt the optimistic view that this situation has been frequent in the history of medicine and that treatments may become available in the future.[1]

3

BRIEF HISTORICAL PERSPECTIVE

Most fetal investigation techniques were developed in the 1960s and 1970s. They can be classified into two main groups: in the first group images from ultrasound are produced and interpreted, and in the second group a biological sample has to be taken and analysed (amniotic liquid, placenta, fetal blood or tissue, maternal blood). In both groups, the types of fetal conditions identified will be presented in a chronological order based on stage of development.

The following summary could lead the reader to believe that current techniques are fully scientifically validated after many decades of research. In reality, they are still criticised and modified in the hope of improving their performances and decreasing their negative effects. Since the emergence of these techniques, the same trends have been in progress: researchers and industrial sponsors try to get better detection rates of abnormalities, decrease the rate of false-positive results (fetuses wrongly identified as at higher risk of abnormality) and decrease the risks that are associated with the use of the techniques for pregnant women and their fetuses. Another trend is to modify the techniques in order to make the diagnosis of fetal conditions earlier in pregnancy, for instance by taking the sample earlier or decreasing the time that is needed to get the results of the tests.

Investigations based on ultrasound scan

Ultrasonography was derived from the sonar, a technique first used in the maritime field to measure distances under water using sound waves. Between the two World Wars, ultrasound was used in medicine with a therapeutic aim, for instance to destroy tissues in neurosurgery. After the Second World War it was used as a diagnostic tool to examine various pathologies, including brains lesions and breast pathologies.[2]

Ultrasonography was used for the first time in obstetrics by Ian Donald in Scotland at the end of the 1950s.[3] At that time radiological examination of the fetus was used to identify only the bone structure of the fetus. The dangerous consequences of ionising radiations for the fetus led to this method being abandoned and ultrasonography being adopted on a large scale. By the 1960s transabdominal, transvaginal and transrectal scanners were used. The first images were difficult to interpret because of their poor quality. However, ultrasonographers could already diagnose pregnancy failure, evaluate multiple gestations, determine amniotic fluid volume and localise placentae.

Soon after, ultrasonography was also used to detect fetal malformation. The first diagnosis of hydrocephaly was documented in 1961 and anencephaly in 1964. These diagnoses were made in the third trimester of pregnancy and resulted in fetal death. The technique only identified fetuses which would miscarry anyway. This first stage was followed by technical improvements and the advent of more experienced ultrasonographers in the 1970s. This enabled diagnosis to be made in the second trimester. Anencephaly was identified in 1972 by Stuart Campbell in England and spina bifida in 1975, the first cases allowing termination of pregnancy.

Ultrasonography was also progressively used to evaluate fetal growth. In 1969 the first biparietal diameter growth curve was developed in Scotland and is considered as the beginning of fetal biometry.[2] Numerous growth charts based on the measurement of various parts of the fetus have been constructed since. They are used to evaluate whether fetal growth is steady and satisfying and to precisely assess the date of gestation and delivery. The latter assessment reduces rates of induction of labour for post-term pregnancy.[4]

Advancements in electronic and microprocessor technology in the 1980s and 1990s led to an increase in the number of abnormalities that could be identified and the ability to detect them earlier in pregnancy. In the second half of the 1980s Benacerraf, a North American ultrasonographer, identified fetuses at high risk of chromosome abnormalities, for instance Down's syndrome, at 15–20 weeks of pregnancy.[3] The main markers are nuchal-fold thickness, short femur and renal pelvic dilatation. In 1992 diagnosis of fetal trisomies was made in the first trimester of pregnancy—between 11 and 14 weeks—by Nicholaides in the UK. The number of abnormalities visible in the first trimester increased in the latter half of the 1990s, with the advent of the high-resolution scanners. Spina bifida can be detected, as well as some cardiac anomalies, with the emergence of Doppler interrogation of intra-cardiac flow. Doppler ultrasound has also been progressively used to diagnose women at risk of pre-eclampsia and utero-placental arterial compromise, leading to effective therapeutic intervention. The most recent innovations are three-dimensional and four-dimensional ultrasonography.

The detection rate of ultrasonography depends on the abnormalities that are looked for. It also depends on the type of machines used, the experience of the ultrasonographer and some characteristics of the pregnant woman, such as her weight. Despite its limitations the predictive power of ultrasonography is strongly relied on by health practitioners in antenatal care. This method of investigation gives the feeling of opening the 'black box' and making the fetus visible. Its usefulness is not contested, even if there are still some questions about possible long-term fetal risks linked to its repeated use. As a result, ultrasonography is now used on a large scale in industrialised countries. The first routine fetal scan programmes were implemented in Sweden in the 1970s.[3] They spread in industrialised countries in the 1980s. The 20 weeks scan has been a standard practice since the 1990s.[2] However, there are important differences among countries regarding the number of routine scans per pregnancy. Ultrasonography is often used to complement other fetal investigation techniques, that are based on the analysis of maternal or fetal samples (see Box 1.1). These are discussed in subsequent chapters.

Box 1.1 Relationship between the techniques

- The various fetal investigation techniques can be complementary. For instance, ultrasonography gives a precise knowledge of the date of the conception, which allows for a more precise risk estimate by biochemical tests.
- These techniques are also sometimes in competition. Ultrasonography may be used as a diagnostic test to identify some conditions, such as cardiac malformations or neural tube defects. In the USA and UK fewer amniocenteses are performed for neural tube defects because of improved safer detection by ultrasonography.

Investigations based on analysis of a fetal or maternal sample

Amniocentesis

Amniocentesis consists of taking a sample of amniotic fluid and was first used for therapeutic reasons. Tapping of amniotic fluid, or transabdominal amniocentesis, was first reported in the 1880s as a technique for amniotic fluid drainage in cases of polyhydramnios.[4]

In 1956 Fuchs and Riis in Copenhagen used amniocentesis to determine the fetal sex, based on the presence or absence of the Barr body. From the first half of the 1960s onwards, birth of fetuses with sex-linked disorders, such as haemophilia A and Duchenne muscular dystrophy, could be avoided by abortion of male fetuses, since only males can possibly be affected by these pathologies.[2]

Amniocentesis is now used for chromosome analysis, or karyotype, of amniocytes in amniotic fluid. This technique was developed when cytogeneticists could show the chromosomal basis of some abnormalities. In making blood karyotypes, the Frenchman Jerome Lejeune proved in 1959 that 'mongolians' had three chromosomes 21, hence the name of trisomy 21. Karyotypes of amniotic cells allowed Valenti in the USA to report the first diagnosis of fetal Down's syndrome in 1968.[4] Other chromosomal abnormalities can also be diagnosed: for example, trisomy 13 and 18 and sex chromosome abnormalities, like Turner's syndrome and Klinefelter's syndrome. The use of fetal karyotype has dramatically increased since because this test can determine with certainty whether there is a fetal chromosomal abnormality.

In the 1960s amniocentesis was also used to assess the severity of fetal rhesus isoimmunisation by measurement of the yellow pigment bilirubin in the amniotic fluid. The treatment for this was an early induced delivery and blood transfusions of the newborn. In the 1970s fetal blood sampling was also introduced to test the severity of rhesus isoimmunisation. At the same time another use for amniocentesis was discovered: biochemical substances can be measured in the fetal fluid to identify some fetal conditions. In 1972 David Brock in Scotland detected spina bifida and anencephaly by measuring the alpha-fetoprotein (AFP) levels in amniotic fluid at 17 weeks of pregnancy

From the 1980s onwards, the range of fetal conditions amenable to detection by amniocentesis widened. Cells in the amniotic fluid can be analysed not only with cytogenetic and biochemical tools but with molecular biology as well. This allows for the identification of fetal genes (fetal genotype) in the amniotic cells. Recombinant deoxyribonucleic acid (DNA) techniques can now identify many genetic diseases, such as X-linked muscular dystrophy, cystic fibrosis, haemophilia, Huntington's chorea and fragile X syndrome. The number of disorders amenable to DNA analysis is increasing.

Technical improvements, such as the ultrasound guidance of amniocentesis from the 1970s on, and experience gained by obstetricians allowed for a reduction in the drawbacks of the sampling technique. Its use is now safer for fetuses and pregnant women because the risks of induced miscarriage and maternal infection have decreased. However, taking a sample in the second trimester still presents many disadvantages for its users. If there is an abnormality, the diagnosis is made comparatively late. The waiting period before the result is available is also long due to the necessity of culturing the fetal amniotic cells for about 2 weeks. Some researchers tried to alleviate these problems by taking the sample earlier in pregnancy. The first amniocentesis was traditionally made between the 14th and 17th weeks. In 1988 Benacerraf conducted an amniocentesis between the 11th and 14th weeks in the USA. The high incidence of fetal loss, however, makes this practice not very popular. In an attempt to get quicker results, new laboratory techniques have been implemented. Fluorescence in situ hybridisation (FISH) allows for a rapid chromosomal analysis of uncultured amniotic fluid cells (24–48 hours), but identifies a more limited number of chromosomal abnormalities.

Chorionic Villus Sampling—placental biopsy

In the 1970s chorionic villus sampling (CVS) was developed simultaneously in many countries. It is a biopsy of the placenta in early pregnancy through the uterine cervix or maternal abdomen. As early as the 1970s the ultrasonographic guidance of the sampling was introduced and this made the procedure less dangerous for the fetus. The first characteristics that CVS could identify were fetal sex and haemoglobinopathies, and then it widened to all the fetal pathologies that can be detected with a chromosomal, biochemical or genetic analysis. CVS is, for instance used to diagnose genetic inherited conditions such as cystic fibrosis, myopathy, thalassaemia and sickle-cell anaemia.

The increase in its use is due to the earlier timing of the procedure compared to amniocentesis. It can be performed after 10 weeks of pregnancy. Another reason for the success of CVS technique is the speed of the diagnosis. It offers the possibility of obtaining a karyotype after 3–4 hours, with confirmation in 24–48 hours, because the cells in the sampled tissues are proliferating.[5] However, this analysis on direct preparation or short-term culture is prone to false-positive and false-negative results. Many laboratories prefer to culture the cells, even though the results take about 2 weeks,[4] and the risk of maternal cell contamination is higher.[5] Another drawback of this procedure is the risk of induced miscarriage that is sometimes reported to be higher than for amniocentesis.

Fetoscopy

In the early 1970s this technique was implemented for direct visualisation of the fetus and its spine with a probe (fibreoptic endoscope) introduced into the uterus through the abdominal wall. It allowed the identification of dysmorphic features. It was progressively replaced by ultrasonography following improvements in the latest performances. This procedure has been almost abandoned now because the visual field is very limited and the risks of fetal loss are high.

Since then fetoscopy has been used to help particular sampling techniques. Due to a high rate of fetal loss and amniotic fluid leak, fetoscopic blood sampling was progressively replaced in the 1980s by CVS and cordocentesis.

Fetal Blood Sampling (FBS)

The first large series of cordocentesis for FBS came from France in 1983, where it was used to detect haemophilia A in utero.[2] A sample of fetal blood is taken, most of the time from the umbilical cord, with a needle that is passed through the maternal abdominal wall under ultrasonographic guidance. It is usually performed at 18–21 weeks of gestation. Fetal blood can also be sampled from the intrahepatic portion of the umbilical vein.

Cordocentesis allows direct estimation of fetal haemoglobin, bilirubin and other parameters. Blood samples may also be used to make a karyotype or a DNA analysis. It also permits the detection of immunodeficiencies, like fetal isoimmunisation, heritable blood disorders (such as thalassaemia and haemophilia), metabolic disorders, chromosomal abnormalities, intrauterine growth retardation and fetal infections (toxoplasmosis, rubella, cytomegalovirus, varicella-zoster). However, the frequency of the use of cordocentesis is declining because of the level of fetal loss. It is being replaced by DNA analysis of cells from chorionic villi or amniotic fluid to diagnose haemophilia, haemoglobinopathies and fetal infections. The major indication in current clinical practice is for pregnancies where a rapid diagnostic result is needed. Results of karyotypes, for instance, are available in 48–72 hours by culture of lymphocytes. Since the late 1980s this technique of aspiration with ultrasound guidance has also been used to sample fetal tissues other than blood, such as liver, skin, muscle, tumour biopsy or fluid.

The various techniques of sampling and analysing the samples that have been presented here are diagnostic tests. They give a definitive result, but carry a risk of pregnancy loss, by inducing miscarriage, preterm labour or intrauterine fetal death. Very occasionally they may also carry a risk of maternal infection. They need to be performed by highly skilled staff and are expensive. In order to select pregnancies that may be at higher risk of fetal problems and would require a diagnostic test, screening tests based on biological samplings have been developed, termed maternal serum markers.

Maternal serum markers

This procedure consists of the analysis of biochemical markers by measuring hormone levels in maternal serum or a blood sample. It was discovered that alpha fetoprotein (AFP) rate in amniotic fluid was higher in case of fetal neural tube defect—spina bifida and anencephaly—causing some biomedical researchers to look for the same substance in maternal blood.[2] In 1973, the Scot David Brock showed that the AFP level in maternal serum was unusually high when the fetus was affected with a neural tube defect. These levels could also be higher in cases of multiple pregnancies, pregnancies complicated by bleeding and intrauterine growth retardation. At the end of the 1970s, the first programme for prenatal screening of spina bifida by measurement of AFP level in maternal serum was implemented in Scotland.[2]

The samples that were obtained in the screening programmes for neural tube defects were used for retrospective biochemical analysis. The researchers measured various blood substances and combined these results with information about the health of the newborn. In 1984 in the USA Merkatz found a link between fetal Down's syndrome and low AFP level at 16th week of gestation. This discovery was also made by Cuckle and Wald in the UK at nearly the same time. At the end of the 1980s other single markers for Down's syndrome were found. Tests were developed with a combination of markers in increasing numbers to improve the detection rate and decrease the false-positive rate. This is discussed in more detail in Chapter 9. Scientific controversies on the advantages and limits of these various tests have always been important.[6] However, the benefits of these screening tests were considered important and the first screening programmes for fetal Down's syndrome in low-risk populations were implemented in industrialised health systems in the beginning of the 1990s. In the mid 1990s these programmes spread in Europe and UK.

The search for better performances of Down's syndrome biochemical tests led to their use with ultrasound. Fetal scans allow for a more precise knowledge of the duration of pregnancy and this improves the accuracy of the risk calculation of the biochemical test. Moreover, the results from both screening tests can be combined (see Ch. 7). With the advent of earlier screening tests and rapid analysis, screening tests can be performed and reported on the same day. The risk estimate is immediately calculated and communicated to the pregnant women, all within a 1-hour visit to a multidisciplinary one-stop clinic.[19] If the screening test indicates that the woman is at higher risk, the sampling for the karyotype may be organised quickly. This procedure raises some controversies as well because the very quick delivery of the result to pregnant women may not give them time to consider the ramifications of the diagnostic test. In the future some researchers suggest that they could identify circulating fetal cells or DNA from maternal blood to diagnose Down's syndrome.

POLICY AGENDA FOR SCREENING AND EMERGING ROLES

In industrialised countries, the implementation of antenatal screening and diagnostic programmes has often preceded the intervention of decision makers and the emergence of a public debate about their social impact and associated ethical problems. In Europe and the UK, these programmes emerged locally on the initiatives of innovators who introduced experimental techniques with research monies.[8] These have progressively been offered to pregnant women on a local basis and were discussed in health practitioners' circles and the media. Policy makers then intervened to regulate the use of the techniques and solve the following problems: safety of these techniques for fetuses and pregnant women, control of the quality of the examination results, inequalities of access in various parts of the country, and how to pay for these developments if their access and use were to be widened in the public sector of health systems. The types of screening programmes that are funded with public money are very variable in industrialised countries. A few, such as Ireland, did not implement any screening programme for chromosomal and genetic abnormalities. Some, such as Japan and the Netherlands,[9] set severe limits to screening programmes.

The organisation of mass screening programmes for fetal abnormalities is often very complex, reflecting the various political, economical and professional interests involved. The example of Down's syndrome screening implementation in the UK sheds light on the broader context of the use of fetal investigation techniques. In the 1970s diagnostic techniques—amniocentesis and CVS—were implemented in the National Health Service (NHS) following local initiatives with an overlap between research and service provision. The techniques used and access to these local programmes varied considerably. The same heterogeneity was observed at the end of the 1980s and the 1990s, when biochemical tests and ultrasound scans were

implemented in the NHS on a local basis. Patchy service provision and lack of agreement about the best test to use have been criticised in biomedical circles and some media, but there was not much public discussion about the social impact of prenatal screening. Some psychologists and sociologists raised concerns about lack of adequate counselling of pregnant women (see below). A few committees on bioethics and genetics wrote reports about prenatal screening and placed emphasis on respect for patient autonomy.

The Department of Health has intervened to regulate the quality of the activity, to address concerns about the ad hoc provision of services and to develop national standards. It created a network of national, regional and local coordinators in December 2000 under the auspices of the UK National Screening Committee (NSC). Many of these coordinators are midwives. They were commissioned to monitor antenatal screening tests, standardise screening services between various local providers, improve the collaboration between clinicians in primary care and hospitals and provide training for community midwives and hospital staff. The UK Government announced a Down's syndrome Screening Programme in 2001 and provided a budget for it. The decision to set standards avoided a difficult decision about methods but also stimulated considerable debate and competition among British research teams developing various tests.[10] The NSC establishes new guidelines on a regular basis to take into account the latest scientific innovations. However, implementation of these standards remains variable.

THE SOCIAL IMPACT OF ANTENATAL TESTING

The introduction of fetal investigation techniques has led to social and economical changes in the organisation of health systems and biomedical industries in industrialised countries. It also has serious ethical and social consequences (see Box 1.2) and has modified pregnant women's experiences and expectations of antenatal care and pregnancy.

Box 1.2 Ethical and social consequences of prenatal screening

- Some stakeholders state that fetal investigation techniques lead to a new form of eugenics.
- The question of the impact on disabled people and their relatives has been raised.
- Their introduction modified health practitioners' tasks.

Changes in the organisation of healthcare systems

In many industrialised countries increasing budgets have been dedicated to implementing fetal investigation techniques. In teaching hospitals, prenatal testing led to the creation of cytogenetics laboratories and clinical genetics services from the 1970s, ultrasound departments from the 1980s, and additional activities for biochemical laboratories from the 1990s. Techniques like ultrasound, amniocentesis, CVS and biochemical tests spread into the private healthcare sector of many countries as well.

Research activities on prenatal testing developed mainly in public hospitals. They led to the growth of a new sector of the biomedical industry. North American, Japanese and European firms contributed to produce products, such as ultrasound scanners, biochemical analysers, chemical reagents and software. Some researchers took out patents on their innovations, for instance on software for risk estimates for biochemical tests in the UK.

Implementation of fetal investigation techniques also led to changes in the organisation of the professions that specialised in prenatal care. New tasks and opportunities arose for the established professions of obstetricians and midwives, such as the post of screening coordinator and fetal medicine sub-specialists. In addition, a new occupation emerged mainly due to prenatal testing: ultrasonographers. They are recruited from radiologists, obstetricians, gynaecologists and midwives. In the past, ultrasonography had little quality control, especially when professions started to use fetal ultrasound scans without any specific training and utilisation of the technique without training was

identified as a problem. The emergence of this technique also modified the relationship between prenatal health practitioners. Ultrasonographers became indispensable colleagues to obstetricians, midwives and general practitioners.

In some countries the changes brought about by the emergence of fetal investigation techniques went beyond the occupational milieu. Users' groups have been established to support pregnant women in their decision making related to prenatal testing and after termination for fetal abnormality. Some associations predated prenatal tests whilst others formed specifically to address issues surrounding these tests. They usually have a help line, a web site and provide pregnant women with written information. Volunteers can become professionalised and develop knowledge and contact networks in prenatal care institutions, in order to answer to the questions of pregnant women.

Ethical questioning and debates on eugenics

Prenatal testing sometimes leads to abortion due to fetal abnormality or to procedure-induced miscarriage. Practices may be considered morally legitimate so long as the fetus is not considered as a living being. This hypothesis is disputed by various stakeholders. Some religious authorities, especially Catholic ones, condemn abortion as immoral, even for therapeutic reasons. They declare that the embryo is not just a complex of organs and tissues in the womb of a woman but the product of the creative intention of God, and a human person from the time of conception onwards. According to them, use of fetal investigation techniques is moral only if the methods employed safeguard the life and integrity of the embryo and the mother [11] Some pro-life groups voice a strong opposition to termination of abnormal fetuses as well, but others are favourable to it.

Promoters of prenatal diagnosis argue that medical abortion for fetal abnormalities is a legitimate practice so long as the screening service is based on the informed choice of pregnant women.[12] This model of individual choice and consumer demand is based on a right that women have gained: the right to own and control their own bodies, including the right to choose to abort.[13] Advocates of prenatal diagnosis emphasise that this right is all the more important to women as they are usually the ones who have to bring up children and care for disabled and sick people in contemporary society.[14]

Some philosophers and sociologists question this view and argue that choosing whether to have a child is different from choosing the characteristics of a fetus.[15,16] It reveals a conditional attitude towards children and parenting that is morally questionable.[17] In addition, selective termination falls within the scope of eugenics, that is the search for an improvement of the human gene pool by the prevention of the birth of some individuals whose life is considered not worth of living.[15,16] These practices are not imposed in an authoritarian way by the governments of democratic societies. It can be regarded as 'back door eugenics', left to the free choice of parents, and resting on the individual search for an healthy child. It can be argued that this is encouraged by health practitioners.[13,15]

However, the use of the term 'eugenics' raises many controversies. Some social scientists argue that this word has too indeterminate a meaning and too many negative historical connotations to be applied to the current situation in a non-polemical way.[18] Some clinicians explain that parents who choose not to have a disabled child do not intend to improve the genetics of the population, nor harm disabled people, but do so because they anticipate the complex needs of severely disabled children will have major implications for the financial situation and quality of life of their families.

Some disabled activists argue that not only parents, but also governments, have eugenic intentions in so far as most prenatal screening programmes are state-funded.[19] They interpret this as a collective will to decrease the number of disabled people in order to economise on the expenditure on their social and health care. As there is no objective way to decide whether prenatal screening is cost-beneficial to society as a whole, it has been suggested that prenatal screening and diagnostic tests should be funded by parents.[20] However, this could create an economic barrier to access.

What level of fetal abnormality and—when the diagnosis is uncertain—what likelihood of disability justifies termination of pregnancy? Surprisingly, advocates and opponents of prenatal testing raise

these similar concerns about the so-called 'slippery slope'. Some health practitioners feel that it would be wrong to comply with the requests of parents who ask for termination on account of minor abnormalities. Some parents have the feeling that the responsibility of this decision should be left to them.

It is also feared that an increasing number of abortions could be requested for common characteristics such as fetal sex. Fetal investigation techniques permit the identification of fetal sex. In countries such as China and India, abortions of female fetuses led to an important imbalance in the sex ratio of the population. According to some feminist sociologists, fetal investigation techniques may be used to discriminate against women and ethnic minorities in industrialised countries.[21,22] Others wonder why health practitioners accept abortions on the grounds of disability and not fetal sex. Promoters of prenatal diagnosis reply that disability is a source of suffering and illness that is not comparable with suffering associated with gender.[13]

Activists and theorists of disability are concerned about the increasing number of abortions for potential abnormality. They fear that budgets dedicated to health, social and educative care for disabled people will be reduced, as a decrease in their number is anticipated in industrialised countries. A substantive reduction in the number of people born with some chromosomal and genetic abnormalities has already been observed. In various local screening programmes implemented in 10 industrialised countries, an average of 50% of Down's syndrome fetuses—the most frequent genetic abnormality—have been prenatally diagnosed and terminated.[23] In Greece the number of people born with thalassaemia has decreased by 90% in the 1990s.[9] However, the total number of disabled people will certainly not diminish in industrialised countries. Many impairments are acquired during life and the increasing life span increases their number.[14] Moreover, neonatal resuscitation units allow some premature babies with heavy physical and mental disabilities to survive. Some disability activists argue that budgets for prenatal screening would be better used to improve the social integration of disabled people.

Their other concern is the consequence of the existence of prenatal testing for the public image of disabled people. The general public and practitioners in prenatal care often lack any practical experience of people with mental and physical disabilities and hold an over-pessimistic view of them.[24] Disabled people are often perceived as suffering individuals, always depending on others and unable to have a social life, even if these stereotypes are contradicted in the literature written by disabled people and their relatives. It is feared that people living with congenital abnormalities that can be detected prenatally, such as Down's syndrome, could be even more stigmatised in the future as 'failures' of preventive medicine.

For some sociologists prenatal testing reinforces the trend already perceptible in the 'medical model' of disability, which states that the problems of disabled people and their relatives come from the biological impairment of the individual. An opposite 'social model' can be developed: the difficulties of disabled people may come less from their own impairment than from the discriminations and stigmatisations they experience in contemporary society.[13,17,25] This can be observed in the fields of work, school, health, housing, leisure, etc. It has been argued that prenatal tests individualise the reasons for fetal abnormalities, putting responsibility on the pregnant woman or the couple.[26] According to some social scientists, instead of changing the society to adapt it to disabled people, one chooses to prevent the birth of disabled people.

Changes in the practices of health practitioners

The emergence of fetal investigation techniques has greatly changed clinical practices. Tests are able to identify many health problems of fetuses and pregnant women. Usually they show that fetal development is normal, which is reassuring for pregnant women and practitioners.

However, some health professionals are unhappy with these changes in antenatal care. Routine prenatal screening is much criticised. Some clinicians refrain from participating in abortion operations on moral grounds and are unhappy to take part in abortion-orientated prenatal diagnostic procedure. Others feel that fetal investigation techniques represent scientific and medical progress but complain that they don't have enough technical and human

resources to implement them appropriately. Techniques change so rapidly that front-line practitioners in maternity units cannot always provide what they feel would be the best screening facilities for pregnant women. Human resources may also be insufficient. According to some surveys carried out in the UK, many midwives and obstetricians are unhappy with the lack of time and resources for counselling.[27,28] They have difficulties in keeping up to date with new prenatal diagnostic procedures and emphasise the complexities of assessing pregnancy risk. The communication with pregnant women may be difficult due to the probabilistic nature of the information and the complexity of all the technical options available at various times in pregnancy. They have to present all pregnant women with the implications of fetal abnormalities with very low probability of occurence, which may potentially distress an entire population. If they fail to do so, not providing the information precludes informed choice.[29] Techniques for presenting this information are presented in Chapter 2.

Some clinicians believe that the public's expectations of screening may be unrealistically high.[4] The public may think that all abnormalities can be detected, or may not realise that affected cases are missed even when that condition is being screened for. Health practitioners fear the legal proceedings that parents could start after the birth of a child with an abnormality. In the USA some litigations concerning 'wrongful birth' became famous.[30] As a result, many clinicians may practise 'defensively' to avoid litigation. They employ all possible screening and diagnostic technologies to avoid being accused of professional failure. In industrialised countries a few legal cases have placed pressure on the health systems to use screening tests as often as possible rather than proceeding with caution.[31]

Impact on women's experiences of pregnancy

The development of fetal investigation techniques falls within the framework of a general trend towards medicalisation of pregnancy and reproduction that started with the development of obstetrics. Pregnant women and their relatives currently have the opportunity to reduce the probability of having a child with some abnormal characteristics.

Advocates of prenatal screening and diagnosis emphasise the demand of pregnant women and the general public for these tests. The percentages of pregnant women who accept or refuse the principle and the use of prenatal tests have important political significance. Public authorities in most industrialised countries funded mass screening programmes because of the supposed will of pregnant women to use prenatal tests. However, it is likely that this supposition has no clear basis, due to the variety of female opinions about this. Attitudes vary from one group to another and some individuals may be in favour of one technique but opposed to another. Sociologists have shown the variety of women's attitudes towards prenatal testing depending on factors such as their social background, religious or moral beliefs, previous experiences, attitudes of partner or relatives, etc.[33]

According to proponents of prenatal diagnosis, the popularity of the tests is mainly due to their capacity to reassure individuals who feel psychologically or economically unable to bring up a disabled child. They also argue that tests allow parents who already have a child with a chromosomal or genetic condition to start another pregnancy avoiding the possibility of having another child with that condition. However, critics emphasise that these parents may be ambivalent towards the tests and prefer not to start another pregnancy because using the tests would devalue their existing child.

The anguish of pregnant women before and after having the tests

In contrast to arguments about reassurance, psychologists and sociologists have shown that prenatal tests often have negative psychological side effects. According to Katz-Rothman,[32] screening procedures changed the experience of pregnancy because they influenced the mother–fetal relationship. Pregnant women may live a 'tentative pregnancy'. They don't bond with their baby until they have been told that the results of the tests are fine. They may, for instance, not acknowledge that early 'flutterings' are fetal movements.

Decision making concerning prenatal tests may be agonizing. In some cases risks linked to the diagnostic procedure are bigger than the estimated risk of abnormality in the fetus. For instance, when the

biochemical screening test for Down's syndrome indicates a risk of 1 in 250, a diagnostic test such as a karyotype with amniocentesis is offered. The risk of fetal loss induced by this procedure is generally considered to be 1 in 100.

The diagnosis of fetal abnormality is still more agonizing. It is then the responsibility of the pregnant woman to decide whether the fetus has the right to enter into the human community or not. Choosing to end a wanted pregnancy after a positive diagnosis is painful and creates long-term psychological sequelae.[33] Making the decision is still more difficult when the likelihood of disability associated with the diagnosis is not precisely known. The 'difficult-to-be-sure-what-will-happen diagnosis' generates much anxiety in parents. This is exposed in more detail in Chapter 3.

Pregnant women may also be distressed by wrong results of screening or diagnostic tests. The anguish created by a false-positive result in a screening programme is not easy to forget, even after receiving a reassuring diagnostic test result.[32,34] False-negative results of screening also have worrying consequences because women are precluded from undergoing a diagnostic test. This often leads to anger and frustration in mothers and their relatives after the birth. Psychologists argue that these parents have higher parenting stress and more negative attitudes towards their children than parents not offered a test or those who declined a test.[35]

The anxiety, or even anguish, felt by pregnant women negatively affects their ability to make decisions about the future of their fetus. In principle, screening and diagnostic tests are recommended by health practitioners and used with the informed consent of the pregnant woman. As a rational human being, a woman is supposed to be able to decide whether the test is useful for her and her fetus or not. Women have to choose between the risk of having a disabled child and risks associated with diagnostic procedures.

Psychologists and sociologists argue that this model is over rationalistic and does not take into account the practical conditions of the tests.[36–38] In practice women may be uncertain about their own preferences and unable to make a well thought out choice when asked to decide quickly in a stressful situation. Women often do not have enough information about prenatal tests, their implications or the conditions that are looked for. Research has shown that a sizeable minority of women were uncertain or incorrect in identifying which tests they had undergone in a recent pregnancy.[39–41] For instance, when undergoing routine screening, women are often knowledgeable about practical aspects of screening tests, but lack information about the likelihood and implications of possible results and often don't understand the meaning of a false-positive or a false-negative result.

Organisational and professional factors appear to limit the ability of women to make informed choices. Their poor knowledge of prenatal tests often reflects the poor quality of information they get from health professionals. The routine nature of tests such as maternal serum tests and ultrasound scans lead women to think that these tests are just another part of the usual package of prenatal care, that they have been scientifically validated as the best procedures to follow to ensure the health of the fetus, and that there is no active decision to be made. It has been shown in the UK that routine screening tests for Down's syndrome may be presented in such a way as to encourage women to undergo the test.[42] A strong pro-testing institutional culture has led to women's high level of maternal serum test acceptance.[37] Ultrasonography is another technique that pregnant women often do not know much about. They may be unaware of the abnormalities that can be detected or even unaware that abnormalities are being looked for. When an abnormality is identified, parents are faced with results and decisions for which they are unprepared.

To solve these problems professional guidelines recommend that health practitioners work in a non-directive way. However, this principle is difficult to apply in daily practice and practitioners sometimes have doubts about whether it could be achieved.[43] Some women ask for direct guidance: 'What would you do ?' Clinicians sometimes admit that they make the decision for the woman, either covertly or overtly, in her 'best interests'.[44] In making the decision they take the burden of responsibility and guilt away from the pregnant woman. In the 1980s, some British obstetricians strongly recommended to terminate a pregnancy if it was found to show any abnormality and provided amniocentesis only on condition that the woman

first agreed to an abortion of an affected fetus.[36] Current studies report more subtle forms of imposition of prenatal tests. In deciding what information is needed and how to present it, health practitioners may strongly reduce the margin of manoeuvre of pregnant women.[43] This slippage between choice and coercion may happen even when clinicians use all the vocabulary of informed consent. In emphasising potential benefits of screening to the neglect of potential harms, midwives may lead women to accept prenatal tests.[45]

CONCLUSION

Historical and sociological approaches to fetal investigation techniques show how widespread and nevertheless controversial they are in industrialised countries. Their use and their conceptions are very diverse and this leads stakeholders to hold many opposing views that may paradoxically be all simultaneously true. Some examples of these are shown in Box 1.3.

In such a varied and paradoxical situation, clinicians

Box 1.3 The paradoxes of prenatal screening

- The public's expectations of screening may be unrealistically high AND a vast majority of women are poorly informed about prenatal tests, including tests they had in a recent pregnancy.
- Pregnant women may look for the perfect baby AND poorly informed or indifferent women experience pressures to get tested.
- Pregnant women may be perfectly happy with the screening procedure provided AND some of them experience anguish and long-term psychological trauma in undertaking the tests.
- Clinicians may screen pregnant women systematically to avoid potential lawsuits AND some of them provide a screening service based on personal choice with appropriate information available.
- Health care settings may implement a strongly pro-testing policy AND some of them don't offer some prenatal tests because they lack the technical or human resources needed.
- Fetal investigation techniques are technology push AND consumer pull.

Box 1.3   The paradoxes of prenatal screening—cont'd

who use fetal investigation techniques have the crucial responsibility of giving the possibility of choice to pregnant women. This may be increasingly difficult as prenatal screening expands, as it will still more be perceived as part of the usual standard package of prenatal care. It is essential to adapt the organisation of care to the needs of each pregnant woman, however variable they are: from those who wish to avoid the birth of a disabled child at all cost to those who decline testing as potential abortion. If health practitioners fail to do so, fetal investigation techniques may become an additional method of coercion in modern societies that delude themselves when using the words liberty and choice.

Key Practice Points

■ The development of fetal investigations has changed the face of antenatal care.

■ The way that services are organised impacts on women's ability to make informed choices about antenatal testing.

■ Fetal investigations have developed differently in different countries, depending on social and political pressures.

■ Fear of litigation can make clinicians more likely to instigate prenatal testing.

References

1. Chamberlain G. What is modern antenatal care of the fetus? In: Chamberlain G, ed. Modern antenatal care of the fetus. Oxford: Blackwell; 1990:1–12.
2. Woo J. A short history of the development of ultrasound in obstetrics and gynecology, Part 3. 2001. Online. Available: http://www.obultrasound.net/history3.html
3. Campbell S. History of ultrasound in obstetrics and gynecology. FIGO 2000 Conference. Online. Available: http://www.obgyn.net/avtranscripts/FIGO_historycampbell.htm
4. Rodeck CH, Pandya P. Prenatal diagnosis of fetal abnormalities. In: Chamberlain G, Steer PH, eds. Turnbull's obstetrics. 3rd edn. London: Churchill Livingstone; 2001:169–196.
5. Gosden C, Tabor A, Leck I, et al. Amniocentesis and CVS. In: Wald N, Leck I, eds. Antenatal and neonatal screening. 2nd edn. Oxford: Oxford University Press; 2000:470–516.
6. Reynolds T. Down's syndrome screening: a controversial test, with more controversy to come! J Clin Pathol 2000; 53:893–898.
7. Bindra R, Heath V, Liao A, Spencer K, Nicolaides K. One-stop clinic for assessment of risk for trisomy 21 at 11–14 weeks: a prospective study of 15 030 pregnancies. Ultrasound Obstet Gynecol 2002; 20:219–225.
8. Reid M. The diffusion of four prenatal screening tests across Europe. London: King's Fund Centre; 1991.
9. Petrogiannis K, Tymstra T, Jallinoja P, Ettore E. Review of policy, law and ethics. In: Ettore E, ed. Before birth. Understanding prenatal screening. Aldershot: Ashgate; 2001:38–52.
10. Kerr A. Genetics and society. A sociology of disease. London: Routledge; 2004:74–82.
11. Sutton A. Prenatal diagnosis: confronting the ethical issues. London: The Linacre Centre; 1990:101.
12. Wald N, Leck I, Muyr-Gray J. Ethics of antenatal and neonatal screening. In: Wald N, Leck I, eds. Antenatal and neonatal screening. 2nd edn. Oxford: Oxford University Press; 2000:543–555.
13. Shakespeare T. Choices and rights: eugenics, genetics and disability equality. Disability and Society, 1998; 13(5):665–681.
14. Ash A. Prenatal diagnosis and selective abortions: a challenge to practice and policy. American Journal of Public Health 1999; 89(11):1649–1657.
15. Duster T. Back to eugenics. New York: Routledge; 1990.
16. McNally R. Eugenics here and now. In: Glasner P, Rothman H, eds. Genetic imaginations. Aldershot: Ashgate; 1998.
17. Vehmas S. Live and let die? Disability in bioethics. New Review of Bioethics 2003:1(1):145–157.
18. Paul D. Eugenic anxieties, social realities, and political choices. In: Jacob M, ed. The politics of western science 1640–1990. Atlantic Highlands, NJ: Humanity Books; 1994.
19. Shakespeare T. Losing the plot? Medical and activist discourses of the contemporary genetics and disability. In: Conrad P, Gabe J, eds. Sociological perspectives on the new genetics. Oxford: Blackwell: 1999:171–190.
20. Thornton J. Should health screening be private? Bury St Edmunds: The IEA Health and Welfare Unit, St Edmundsbury Press; 1999.

21. Stacey M. The new genetics: a feminist view. In: Marteau T, Richards M, eds. The troubled helix. Social and psychological implications of the new human genetics. Cambridge: Cambridge University Press; 1996:331–349.

22. Bradby H. Genetics and racism. In: Marteau T, Richards M, eds. The troubled helix. Social and psychological implications of the new human genetics. Cambridge: Cambridge University Press; 1996:295–316.

23. International Clearinghouse for Birth Defects Monitoring Systems. Annual report 2003. Online. Available: http://icbd.org/document/AR2003/p2.pdf

24. Williams C. What constitutes balanced information in the practitioner's portrayals of Down's syndrome? Midwifery 2002; 18(3):230–237.

25. Ash A. Prenatal diagnosis and selective abortions: a challenge to practice and policy. American Journal of Public Health 1999; 89(11):1649–1657.

26. Alderson P. Prenatal screening, ethics and Down's syndrome: a literature review. Nursing Ethics 2001; 8(4):360–374.

27. Fairgrieve S, Magnay D, White I, Burn J. Maternal serum screening for Down's syndrome: a survey of midwives' views. Public Health 1997; 111:383–385.

28. Green J. Serum screening for Down's syndrome; experience of obstetricians in England and Wales. BMJ 1994; 309:769–772.

29. Heyman B, Henriksen M. Risk, age and pregnancy. A case study of prenatal genetic screening and testing. Basingstoke: Palgrave; 2001.

30. Nelkin D, Tancredi L. Dangerous diagnostics: the social power of biological information. New York: Basic Books; 1989.

31. Lupton D. The imperative of health. Public health and the regulated body. London: Sage; 1995:77–103.

32. Katz-Rothman B. The tentative pregnancy. Amniocentesis and the sexual politics of motherhood. London: Pandora; 1988.

33. Rapp R. Testing women, testing the foetus. New York: Routledge; 2000.

34. Green J, Statham H. Psychosocial aspects of prenatal screening and testing. In: Marteau T, Richards M, eds. The troubled helix. Social and psychological implications of the new human genetics. Cambridge: Cambridge University Press; 1996:140–163.

35. Hall S, Bobrow M, Marteau T. Psychological consequences for parents of false negative results on prenatal screening for DS: retrospective interview study. BMJ 2000; 320(7232):407–412.

36. Farrant W. Who's for amniocentesis? The politics of prenatal screening. In: Homans H, ed. The sexual politics of reproduction. Aldershot: Gower; 1985.

37. Press N, Browner CH. Why women say yes to prenatal diagnosis. Social Science and Medicine 1997; 45(7):979–989.

38. Green J, et al. Psychosocial aspects of genetic screening of pregnant women and newborns: a systematic review. Health Technology Assessment 2004; 8(33):1–124.

39. Marteau T, et al. Development of a self-administered questionnaire to measure women's knowledge of prenatal screening and diagnostic tests. Journal of Psychosomatic Research 1988; 32(4/5):403–408.

40. Kidd J, Cook R, Marteau M. Is routine AFP screening in pregnancy reassuring? Journal of Psychosomatic Research 1993; 37(7):717–722.

41. Smith D, Shaw R, Marteau T. Informed consent to undergo serum screening for Down's syndrome: the gap between policy and practice. BMJ 1994; 309:776.

42. Marteau T, Slack J, Kidd J, Shaw R. Presenting a routine test in antenatal care: practice observed. Public Health 1992; 106(2):131–141.

43. Williams C, Alderson P, Farsides B. Too many choices? Hospital and community staff reflect on the future of prenatal screening. Social science and medicine 2002; 55(5):743–753.

44. Williams C, Alderson P, Farsides B. Is nondirectiveness possible within the context of antenatal screening and testing? Social science and medicine 2002; 54:339–347.

45. Pilnick A. Presenting and discussing nuchal translucency screening for fetal abnormality in the UK. Midwifery 2004; 20(1):82–93.

2

Involving parents: information and informed decisions

Amanda Sullivan

INTRODUCTION

. . . I was never told, such and such things we are going to do . . . I was never asked have you any objection to this or that? My will, my wishes, my inclinations were not once consulted . . . I did not find the respect paid usually even to a child . . . the doctors . . . expunged from their conscience all deference to me; giving up so speedily and entirely all attempt at explanation . . .[1]

The above quotation indicates the humiliation felt when professionals do not take the time to explain or discuss plans for care. It is sobering to realise that this was written over 200 years ago when deference to doctors was the cultural norm and there was a view that 'doctor knows best'. The fact that the quotation came from an individual who had been institutionalised and declared 'insane' adds further poignancy. Imagine then how an uninformed mother may feel in today's less deferential information age.

Providing information and involving mothers in decisions about investigations is a vital part of demonstrating respect for those in one's care. For several decades there has been a recognised moral obligation for midwives to provide information and to help mothers make informed choices. That obligation is now included in midwifery's professional regulations.[2] Furthermore, government policy is committed to radically increasing choice within the National Health Service (NHS) and specifically within the maternity services.[3]

This chapter aims to equip midwives with the fundamental knowledge that is needed when helping parents negotiate antenatal investigations. The chapter begins by explaining common terminology associated with antenatal tests. The nature of informed decisions and the midwife's role throughout the testing process are then discussed. Key skills and practice points are also highlighted, in order to help midwives avoid common pitfalls during consultations. Finally, this chapter will consider the midwife's accountability and responsibilities associated with antenatal investigations.

INFORMING THE INFORMERS: COMMON TERMINOLOGY EXPLAINED

Antenatal investigations are performed to provide information that will inform subsequent care. The information may relate to the mother's health and wellbeing, for instance full blood count, blood pressure and urinalysis. Other tests, such as ultrasound anatomy scans, provide information about the baby's development. Sometimes, tests are performed to assess or predict fetal wellbeing. These include ultrasound scans for growth and liquor volume and Doppler assessments. It may be necessary to combine fetal and maternal results to decide the best course of action. The way in which tests are interpreted and acted upon depends upon the reliability of the results. It is essential that midwives can assess test reliability in order to judge how to explain and act on results.

Broadly speaking, tests can be regarded as screening or diagnostic. Screening tests are designed to identify the people who have a high enough risk of a particular disorder to warrant further investigations. For instance, mothers are routinely asked about their previous obstetric history. This is a way of assessing risk for the current pregnancy. If a mother had previously delivered a 4.5 kg baby, it would be worth offering a glucose tolerance test to identify/exclude gestational diabetes. Screening helps to allocate resources to the people most likely to benefit.

Screening for increased risk of a condition requires a different approach than other aspects of midwifery care. In the main, midwives offer care and support in response to a mother's queries or worries. Screening tests are, by definition, applied to an apparently healthy population. The process of informing a mother about her risk of a condition and the options available to her can be more harmful than helpful if handled inappropriately. The benefits of screening should outweigh the harms. Benefits and harms are shown in Figure 2.1.

Midwives play a vital role in delivering the national Antenatal and Newborn Screening Programme. This includes tests for human immunodeficiency virus (HIV), syphilis, hepatitis B, rubella immunity, haemoglobinopathies, Down's syndrome and inborn errors of metabolism such as phenylketonuria. Midwives are responsible for offering,

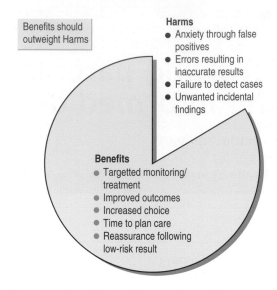

Figure 2.1 Benefits and harms of screening tests.

discussing and performing screening tests and for ensuring that results are communicated and acted upon appropriately. Errors can unfortunately occur at any of these stages, with devastating results. For instance, a mother's date of birth was incorrectly entered onto a Down's syndrome screening request card. This resulted in an inaccurate risk assessment and the subsequent birth of a baby with Down's syndrome. This high-profile case had far-reaching emotional and financial consequences, resulting in a settlement of £500 000.[4] Other programmes, such as breast and cervical screening, have also missed cancers through incorrect analysis of samples.

Since errors in screening can be catastrophic for the public and professionals concerned, the UK National Screening Committee (NSC) was formed to manage the quality and delivery of screening programmes. The Antenatal and Newborn Screening Programme is now overseen by a network of national and regional screening coordinators, many of whom have a midwifery background. Each Trust should also have a local midwifery screening coordinator to act as a specialist resource and to monitor screening within their Trust. These roles were introduced to ensure that quality issues are detected and acted upon in a prompt manner. Screening coordinators also work together with laboratory staff to determine how well screening tests are performing. This includes the number of affected cases detected and the number of false-positive results. Terminology that is commonly used to describe the performance of a test is shown in Box 2.1.

Tests performed by midwives have very different levels of sensitivity and specificity. For instance, HIV testing is very sensitive and specific. Cystic fibrosis screening on the newborn bloodspot test is very sensitive and only misses rare forms of the disease. However, it is not specific to the disorder as it may detect carrier status or appear positive because of meconium contamination on the sample or transient metabolic disturbances (particularly in preterm infants). Down's syndrome screening is currently

---

Box 2.1   Glossary of screening terminology

Sensitivity—this tells you how good a test is at correctly identifying people who have the condition. It is the proportion of people with the condition who are found to be positive on a screening test. This is sometimes referred to as the **detection rate**.

Specificity—this tells you how good a test is at correctly identifying people who do not have the condition. It is the proportion of people who are not affected by a disorder who will be found to be negative on a screening test for that disorder. This is linked to the **true-negative rate**.

Positive predictive value—this is the chance that a positive test result will be correct. In other words, positive predictive value is the proportion of people with a positive result that actually have the condition. This is sometimes referred to as the **odds of being affected given a positive result (OAPR)**.

Negative predictive value—this is the chance that a negative test result will be correct. It is the proportion of people with a negative result that do not have the condition.

False-positive rate—this is the proportion of people who have a positive result but do not have the condition. This is directly related to the specificity or true-negative rate of a test.

False-negative rate—this is the proportion of people who have a negative result but actually have the condition. This is directly related to the sensitivity or detection rate of a test.

---

undertaken with different tests in different parts of the country. Although the NSC have set test performance standards of 75% detection rate for a false-positive rate of 3% or less by April 2007, most areas currently offer tests that do not achieve these standards. Figure 2.2 gives a diagrammatic representation of the specificity of Down's syndrome screening using the triple test. Out of 200 women, an average of 10 receive higher-risk (screen positive) results. However, only around 1 in 60 of those women will actually have a Down's syndrome affected pregnancy. It is also possible that lower-risk (screen negative) women may also have an affected pregnancy.

The NSC also assesses programmes to ensure they do more good than harm at a reasonable cost. There are nationally agreed criteria for screening programmes, as shown in Box 2.2. The next section of this chapter will focus on achieving the final criterion—providing information and facilitating informed decisions.

INFORMED DECISIONS AND THE MIDWIFE'S ROLE

Providing information and helping mothers to decide about their care is fundamental to midwifery practice. The *Midwives' Rules and Standards* state that a midwife *'should enable the woman to make decisions about her care based on her individual needs, by discussing matters fully with her'* (Rule 6, Responsibility and Sphere of Practice p. 16).[2] However, it is not always clear whether women truly make informed decisions or whether they feel adequately prepared to make potentially life-changing decisions. Furthermore, information requirements vary greatly between individuals and situations. The ability to provide the right amount of information in an appropriate manner requires a great deal of perception and self-awareness. Midwives are also sometimes unclear about when to recommend a particular course of action and when to appear neutral, particularly when mothers ask 'What would you do?'

What is an informed decision?

Informed decisions have two important characteristics. First, they must be based on relevant, good-quality information. Second, the decision must

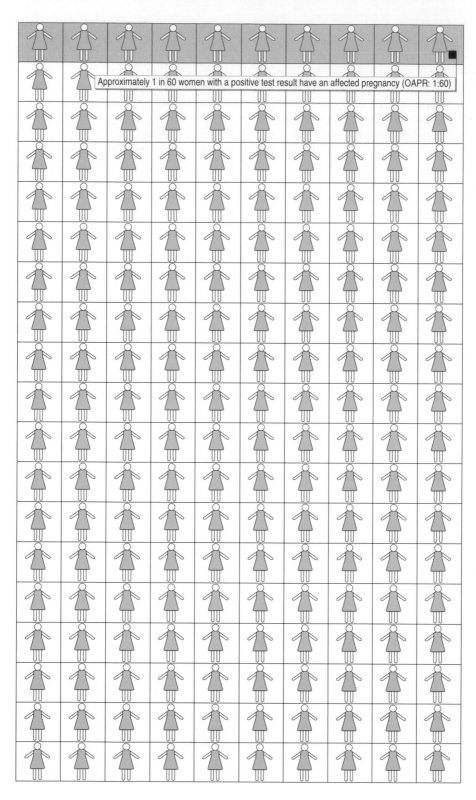

Approximately 1 in 60 women with a positive test result have an affected pregnancy (OAPR: 1:60)

Figure 2.2 200 people.

> **Box 2.2** Summary of the UK National Screening Committee criteria for appraising the viability, effectiveness and appropriateness of a screening programme
>
> **The condition**
> - The condition should be an important health problem.
> - There should be a detectable risk factor, disease marker, latent period or early symptomatic stage.
> - All cost-effective primary prevention should have been implemented.
> - If carriers are identified, the psychological and physical implications should be understood.
>
> **The test**
> - There should be a simple, safe and validated test, with an agreed cut-off.
> - The test should be acceptable to the public.
> - There should be further diagnostic investigations available.
>
> **The treatment**
> - There should be effective treatment available, with evidence that early treatment is more effective than later treatment.
>
> - There should be agreed policies about who should be offered treatment and the appropriate treatment to be offered.
>
> **The screening programme**
> - The programme should reduce mortality or morbidity.
> - Tests that aim to provide information to enable people to make an informed choice (e.g. Down's syndrome screening, cystic fibrosis carrier testing) should accurately measure risk. The information that is provided must be of value and readily understood by the individual being screened.
> - The benefits should outweigh the physical and psychological harm (caused by the test, diagnostic procedures and treatment).
> - There should be agreed quality management standards and quality should be monitored.
> - *Evidence-based information about the consequences of testing and treatment should be available to assist informed choice.*

reflect the decision-maker's values.[5] In order to achieve the first characteristic, midwives must supply the relevant information and ensure that it has been understood. Midwives must also establish the woman's preferences and attitudes towards the test in order to establish whether the decision is informed. This process is sometimes straightforward and takes very little time. For instance, a woman who is offered a test for rubella susceptibility is likely to accept the test as potentially beneficial for present and future pregnancies. Conversely, decisions about fetal anomaly testing can be more complex and can give rise to conflicting values and moral dilemmas. Difficult decisions for the mother require a higher level of skill from the midwife.

The process of making an informed decision can be considered in three main stages.[6] These include:

1. Defining the issue or problem about which a decision needs to be made

2. Giving information about relevant options
3. Deciding on the best course of action.

During a consultation, it is likely that these stages may overlap or be repeated. However, it is useful to consider them separately here, so that decision-making components can be identified and considered in relation to midwifery practice.

Defining the issue

This may be a routine aspect of antenatal care, such as offering a screening test. It may also involve clinical observations or test results. The midwife requires expertise to identify and explain clinical issues. Sometimes, the woman defines an issue, such as reduced fetal movements or concerns about her forthcoming labour. In general, information needs to shared between the midwife and the woman before the issue or problem can be fully defined. This is because the midwife brings a professional perspective to a situation, whilst the mother knows her own priorities and concerns.

This first stage, whereby the decision is defined, is influenced by many factors. Midwives and women bring their own cultural beliefs, attitudes and preferences to a consultation. For instance, most women have views about whether or not they wish to undergo screening for Down's syndrome before this is discussed with a health professional. Box 2.3 gives examples of cultural views and attitudes that women express concerning Down's syndrome. Midwives may also have strong views, although these should not form the basis of recommendations to women.

Although women's views about Down's syndrome and disability in general influence their decisions about Down's syndrome screening, the person offering the test and the way that services are organised are also influential. For instance, a large amount of information is exchanged at the booking visit. It may be the first time that the midwife and mother have met and both may have very little understanding of the other's expectations and priorities. Consequently, mothers may agree to 'conform' to 'routine' care such as ultrasound anomaly scans and hospital delivery without adequate information on which to base their agreement. Indeed, many women may not realise that

---

Box 2.3 Examples of pregnant women's attitudes towards Down's syndrome

- 'I suppose over the years, I've watched programmes about Down's syndrome children and I've seen people cope brilliantly . . . I admire them . . .'
- 'We don't feel we would be strong enough to cope. They say they have quality of life, but to us it would be cruel to let a child suffer . . .'
- 'To us, it's our baby and it will be loved whatever . . .'
- 'I would still love the child, but I would feel sorry for it . . .'
- 'We're not getting any younger and if we weren't here to care for that child, it would be awful. What if the child had to go into a home . . .'
- 'It would be unfair on my other two children . . .'

---

they have a choice in such matters. Where there is a choice, this should be made explicit in verbal and written communications.

Women's views of health professionals in general and the midwife's behaviour are also very important when making decisions. Even when women would like information about investigations, they may be reluctant to seek this from a midwife they perceive to be too busy, unhelpful or unapproachable. This clearly militates against informed decisions. Midwives also influence this stage of decision making by the way that information is portrayed. There are two main psychological mechanisms that midwives should be aware of when explaining a clinical issue:

1. *Framing effects:* The language used to describe a clinical issue affects the way that information is interpreted and perceived. For instance, many women worry about whether they will give birth to a healthy baby. On average, 1 in 50 babies suffer long-term problems. This can sound more worrying than a 2% chance of long-term problems to some parents. A 98% chance of giving birth to a healthy baby seems even more reassuring.

   Midwives frequently give women information about pregnancy-associated risks. This may include the risks of smoking, cot death or breech deliveries. Even when risks are presented in numerical form, their meaning can be distorted. Low probabilities tend to be overweighted and higher probabilities tend to be under-weighted. For instance, most people regard the difference between £10 and £20 to be larger than the difference between £110 and £120. Therefore, care should be taken to present risk information in several ways. For instance, a 1 in 100 risk of a poor outcome should also be presented as a 1% risk or a 99% chance that the risk will not occur.

2. *Order effects*: The order in which information is presented can affect the way that a situation is perceived. Sometimes, the first item may be preferentially retained (primacy effect). Alternatively, the most recent information may be remembered best (recency effect). In practice, this means that it is important that the first and last statements about a topic give the correct

message. For instance, a mother who presents with a small vaginal bleed in early pregnancy should not be greeted with the news that she may be beginning to miscarry. Instead, it is kinder to explain other potential causes before the chances of a miscarriage. Likewise, it can increase distress if the risk of miscarriage is the last message given during a consultation.

In summary, the first stage of informed decision making requires the issue to be defined and mutually understood. Midwives have their own personal and professional perspectives to bring to bear, whilst women will also have a range of expectations and preferences. The way in which midwives present information can greatly affect this stage of decision making. Box 2.4 gives some good practice points to consider when discussing the results of investigations. This is commonly the time when potential problems are identified and subsequent options need to be discussed.

Giving information about relevant options

Midwives are required to perform a delicate balancing act when giving information about different treatment options. Women need the 'right' amount of information to acquire sufficient knowledge without feeling overwhelmed and burdened with the responsibility of choice. But what is the 'right' amount and how should this be delivered? The effectiveness of different strategies in improving decisions is unclear.[7] Choices are also constrained by limited resources or clinical guidelines.

Information should also be evidence-based, but evidence may be limited or apparently conflicting.

Box 2.4 Giving test results: good practice points

State what the results are and what they mean
Establish whether results have been understood
Numbers can be confusing—present them in several ways
Severe anxiety usually arises from misunderstanding
Information about options, verbally and in writing
Timing of results—minimise the period of uncertainty
Invite questions, give contact numbers
Visits are appreciated for face-to-face discussion
Empathy whatever the decision or outcome

Moreover, different 'experts' or professional groups may regard evidence differently. This was highlighted in the high-profile case of Jaymee Bowen, a young girl with leukaemia.[8] Jaymee was refused a second round of NHS treatment on the grounds that she only had a 2% chance of survival. Critics suspected that this decision was taken on the grounds of cost and not because further treatment would prolong her suffering. Following private donation, the doctor who took over her care stated that she belonged to a sub-group of leukaemics with a 30% chance of survival. Jaymee sadly died following the second round of treatment. This section will consider the challenges associated with providing information in relation to midwifery practice. Good practice points will also be identified.

The amount of information that women need varies. Some require detailed information, including rare occurrences, whilst others ask health professionals to make decisions on their behalf. Department of Health guidance recognises that there is always an element of clinical judgement in determining what information to give.[9] However, the presumption should be that women wish to be well informed about different options. Meaningful consent can only be given if the relevant risks and benefits and all options are made clear. If women do not wish to receive such information, this should be clearly documented before investigations are performed. Information giving should be an interactive process, so that the midwife can gauge the woman's existing level of knowledge and understanding, views and information requirements. Inviting women to ask questions helps to guide the consultation in a way that suits women's needs.

Midwives sometimes express concerns about increasing women's knowledge because this also increases anxiety. However, the evidence demonstrates that preparing people for medical interventions is associated with reduced distress.[10] A second misconception is that increasing anxiety is inappropriate, abnormal or undesirable. However, increased anxiety may indicate that individuals are processing information effectively and are actively engaged with the decision-making process. There is some evidence to suggest that this aids long-term coping.[10] It should also be remembered that anxiety is a natural response to stressful and uncertain situations. Information about different treatment options should be seen as distinct from providing information about ways of coping and sources of support.

If choices are limited, it can be difficult to know whether to provide information about *available* options or *all possible* options. For instance, should the option of paying for a test for B Haemolytic Streptococcus carriage be discussed when this is not recommended as a routine screening test? If mothers are told about options they cannot access, this may increase dissatisfaction, whilst failure to disclose other options can deprive mothers of a preferred course of action. Sometimes, information about the reasons for service constraints, such as research evidence of lack of effectiveness, may reduce dissatisfaction. In practice, midwives provide information about additional healthcare options when it is apparent that women would wish to avail themselves of additional facilities. This may include access to independent midwives, National Childbirth Trust classes or private Down's syndrome screening tests.

There are a number of different ways to provide information. Women appreciate honest face-to-face discussion and this should remain the primary source of information. Good quality written information is a useful means of increasing knowledge, but this is only effective if used alongside the opportunity to ask questions and clarify areas of uncertainty. It is also important to provide information in a range of languages, to suit local needs. The availability of written information, particularly for languages other than English, varies considerably from area to area. National resources are increasing. These may eventually replace local initiatives, once standardised screening services are in place.

Parents increasingly obtain information from the internet. However, this does not generally reduce the amount of face-to-face input required. Instead, information obtained from the internet is likely to stimulate more questions and increase the need for discussion. It is therefore essential that midwives are aware of current issues and developments. Some useful sources of information for parents and professionals are shown in Table 2.1. Some of these sites contain information leaflets that can be downloaded and distributed locally. Some are concerned with antenatal investigations in general and some give detailed information about conditions that can be detected. It is likely that a range of health-related information will also become available through videos and interactive television.

Midwives must be able to understand and interpret the evidence base that underpins information about different treatment options. However, journal articles may be biased because research that finds positive effects is more likely to be written up and selected for publication. Midwives often do not have sufficient time or expertise to conduct full literature reviews and critically appraise apparently conflicting studies. However, an increasing number of systematic reviews are now available for clinicians. These reviews extract data from a number of studies and assess overall effectiveness of different treatment options. For instance, the Cochrane Collaboration includes a wide range of reviews on all areas of healthcare, including pregnancy and childbirth. (This is accessible via www.cochrane.org).

Systematic reviews have traditionally focused on evidence from randomised controlled trials. However, systematic methods of reviewing qualitative data, including interviews or observations, are becoming more established. In the practice setting, a simple précis of the main risks and benefits should be presented for all available options. This should be combined with relevant information regarding the mother's situation, views and preferences. In this way, midwives can succeed in providing balanced information that reflects current knowledge but that also takes into account the context of each unique situation. Experienced practitioners may do this intuitively. When information is given about investigations that have demonstrable benefits and very little risk, this can be a very brief process.

In summary, the process of providing information about different options always requires a degree of clinical judgement, but some principles of good practice have been established. The amount of information required is variable and depends on the situation and the individuals concerned. If choices are limited, it is helpful to be honest about this and give rationales where appropriate. Written information is useful to support discussions. Finally, information should be presented in a balanced way.

Deciding on the best course of action

The third stage of decision making involves midwives and parents working together to weigh up all

Table 2.1   Sources of information for professionals and parents

Topic	Source of information	Resources available
Informed Choice leaflets	Midwives Information and Resource Service (MIDIRS) Informed Choice www.infochoice.org	Leaflets to download for parents and professionals. Antenatal topics include alcohol and pregnancy, routine ultrasound scans, screening for congenital abnormalities
Parents' experiences of antenatal screening and diagnosis of fetal abnormality (also includes many other health topics)	DIPEx website www.dipex.org	Parents' experiences and views of the service recorded on video clips and interview transcripts. Includes a range of experiences, including termination of pregnancy
Antenatal screening programmes and standards	National Screening Committee www.nelh.nhs.uk/screening/	National information booklet about Down's syndrome screening to download in a range of languages. Information regarding conditions screened for and current standards
Support for parents making decisions about antenatal testing for the baby	Antenatal Results and Choices (ARC) www.arc-uk.org/	Advice for parents and local contacts. Range of written information leaflets for parents/ grandparents. Information about study days
Neural tube defects	Association of Spina Bifida and Hydrocephalus www.asbah.org	Information leaflets to download. Subjects include anencephaly, hydrocephalus, folic acid in pregnancy, genetic counselling, spina bifida
Patau's syndrome (trisomy 13), Edward's syndrome (trisomy 18) and related disorders (including partial trisomy, mosaicism, rings, translocation, deletion)	Support Organisation for Trisomy 13/18 and Related Disorders (SOFT) www.soft.org.uk/	Support links with other family support, information for parents (free booklet for parents on request)
Haemoglobinopathies	Accessible Publishing of Genetic Information www.chime.ucl.ac.uk/APoGI/	Information on haemoglobinopathies (carrier status and the conditions). Can be downloaded. Includes different couple carrier combinations
Down's syndrome	Down's Syndrome Association (DSA) www.dsa-uk.com/	Information about Down's syndrome and support available when affected children are born
Antenatal screening for fetal abnormality	AnSWeR Antenatal Screening Web Resource http://www.antenataltesting. info/default.html	Ethical dilemmas, experiences of termination of pregnancy and views about disability
Metabolic diseases	Children Living with Inherited Metabolic Diseases (CLIMB) National Information and Advice Centre for Metabolic Diseases www.climb.org.uk	Advice, information and support on all metabolic diseases to children, young adults, families, carers and professionals
Haemoglobinopathy screening	NHS Haemoglobinopathy Screening Programme www.kcl-phs.org.uk/ haemscreening/	Information and policies concerning haemoglobinopathy screening

the options and to choose the best course of action. Although it is important to reach a consensus agreement, the way in which this is achieved inevitably varies according to the individuals involved and the clinical situation. This section outlines key psychological mechanisms that people use for this stage of decision making. It will also provide some examples of different clinical scenarios that require different approaches.

Whilst it is important to work in partnership, women should not be left to make overwhelming decisions without adequate support and guidance. Midwives can provide guidance and influence decisions without being coercive. For instance, when purchasing a new car, most people welcome some guidance and advice even though the final purchase decision is their own. It is customary to give the car salesman an outline specification such as price, size, number of doors and additional extras required. The salesman then gives the choices available that fit the specification. The salesman may then make recommendations in relation to the customer's requirements. This helps the customer decide which car to buy.

It is essential to remember that, when faced with situations in which the outcome is uncertain, people use psychological mechanisms to help them make decisions. Perhaps the most important mechanism is the way that humans reduce complex and unfamiliar information into a format that allows them to make a judgement. We do this by using general rules of thumb or heuristics. In other words, we use previously acquired knowledge to help us understand new information. This is essential for everyday life, but can have negative consequences such as stereotyping or jumping to conclusions.

One commonly used rule of thumb is known as the availability heuristic. In this, an event is viewed as more likely to happen if it is easy to recall an instance of it happening on another occasion. Frequent media reports of adverse events, such as murders, result in a belief that murders are more common than they actually are. Similarly, a woman whose neighbour recently gave birth to a stillborn baby is likely to have a heightened sense of awareness that babies still die unpredictably. She is therefore likely to be more anxious than mothers without exposure to infant mortality. This may

result in a heightened sensitivity to fetal movements and an increased likelihood that she will report reduced fetal movements. In short, previously acquired knowledge impacts on the way that potential problems are identified and on decisions that are made.

Another heuristic that commonly influences decision making is known as the representativeness heuristic. In this, judgements are often made on the basis of previous 'similar cases'. For example, a woman may conclude that she will give birth to a boy because she feels the same as she did in a previous male pregnancy. She may therefore decide to paint the nursery blue and buy blue baby clothes. Midwives also use this heuristic when deciding on the best course of action. This may lead to poor decisions, but can also be regarded as an accumulation of experience that enables clinical judgement. It may be argued that expert decision making encompasses pattern recognition that is recalled subconsciously or intuitively.

Individual beliefs are also very influential when deciding on the best course of action. Many people search for and use evidence in a manner that supports existing beliefs. This means evidence that is consistent with a favoured viewpoint tends to be over-weighted. Unwelcome evidence may be minimised or disregarded. For instance, a mother may justify her decision to continue smoking in pregnancy because her previous baby, with whom she also smoked, was healthy. Similarly, the belief that bad events are more likely to happen to other people in similar circumstances is associated with positive mental health. This is sometimes referred to as a 'warm glow'. Indeed, depressed people are likely to be more realistic about their chances of a risky event occurring.[11]

It is important to bear these mechanisms in mind when women appear to be dismissive of health advice. If this apparent 'denial' puts the mother or baby at risk, it is important to identify misconceptions and challenge these. For instance, the mother who believes it is safe to smoke in pregnancy because her last baby was healthy should be informed that the risks of smoking still relate to the current pregnancy.

It is apparent that a range of psychological mechanisms influence decisions. These mechanisms

Table 2.2 **Different approaches to decision making**

Clinical scenario	Strategies to aid decision making	Midwife's role
Higher-risk Down's syndrome screening result. Can't decide whether to have amniocentesis	Ask mother's worst-case scenario—baby with Down's syndrome or miscarriage of normal baby. Ask what the mother would do in the event of a prenatal Down's syndrome diagnosis (remember that mothers may want a diagnosis for information and not to terminate the pregnancy).	Help mothers understand their options and the potential consequences of each choice. Provide non-judgemental support. Establish mother's views about each potential outcome and the least worse alternative.
Offer of HIV screening test. Mother appears reluctant to have the test	Try to establish reasons for the concerns. Provide information about reduced vertical transmission rates with prophylaxis. Indicate that this is offered routinely and universally. Discuss treatment options if HIV positive.	Inform the mother of the benefits and recommend the test. Identify and correct misconceptions. Acknowledge mother's viewpoint.
'Suspected' breech presentation at 36 weeks. Mother refuses to attend hospital for scan	Explain why it is important to establish the presentation and implications for delivery. Explain options available if breech presentation is confirmed.	Recommend further investigations, whilst acknowledging mother's viewpoint. Emphasise the benefits of pre-labour diagnosis and management plans.

enable us to make sense of and cope with new information. However, it is important for the midwife to recognise when women jump to the wrong conclusions or dismiss health advice. Different situations require different approaches, as shown in Table 2.2. However, decisions should generally involve a level of negotiation, such that the responsibility for the decision is shared.

THE MIDWIFE'S ACCOUNTABILITY AND RESPONSIBILITIES

As stated, informed decisions require the midwife to identify the decision to be made, to discuss available options and then to make a decision in partnership with the woman. Although this process requires a degree of flexibility and clinical judgement, the midwife has a duty of care and has a responsibility to meet certain standards. The *Midwives' Rules and Standards*[2] state that midwives 'should enable the woman to make decisions about her care based on her individual needs, by discussing matters fully with her'. The midwife should also 'respect the woman's right to refuse any advice given' (Rule 6, p. 17). Specific responsibilities in relation to antenatal investigations are listed in Box 2.5. Actions may vary in emergency situations or when the woman does not have the capacity to give consent. Reasons for obtaining and actioning test results may also vary according to local protocols, but the midwife must ensure that this is clear and that mothers know how and when they will receive their results.

Box 2.5   Midwife's role and responsibilities in relation to antenatal investigations

Pre-test responsibilities
- Provide information about the nature and purpose of the test, all available options and common/serious sequelae that may occur as a result of the test
- Include information about benefits and risks
- Give information in a clear and balanced way
- Check that the information has been understood
- Advice must be evidence-based and up-to-date
- Give written information to support discussions
- Give sources of additional information as required
- Document the main points of discussions and advice given
- Document reasons why tests are accepted/declined as discussed
- Document that consent has been obtained (this may be verbal or written)

Performing the test
- Check that the woman understands the reason for testing and the meaning of the results
- Discuss when and how results will be available
- Check how the woman would prefer to receive results (where appropriate)
- Ensure that the request form contains the correct identification and clinical details

- Ensure that tests are only requested when consent has been obtained (some request forms include multiple tests and require unwanted options to be deleted)
- Document that the test has been performed

Post-test responsibilities
- Ensure that investigations ordered by the midwife are reported and actioned appropriately
- Communicate abnormal/equivocal findings to a medical practitioner when a medical opinion is required
- Results should be communicated in a timely, sensitive and comprehensible manner
- Give contact numbers and sources of support when bad news has been portrayed
- Maintain confidentiality, sharing information with other professionals on a need-to-know basis only
- Results should only be discussed with partners/relatives when the mother is also present or has given her express permission
- Document all results and associated discussions
- Results documentation may be in the form of a laboratory report inserted into the notes

---

CONCLUSION

This chapter aims to equip midwives with the knowledge required to help women make informed decisions. When discussing tests, it is essential that the midwife understands the basic principles of each test and can interpret the results. Some basic terminology has been described and this will be applied to specific disorders in subsequent chapters.

Informed decisions are based on good-quality information and reflect the decision-maker's views. The decision-making process is influenced by attitudes, expectations and preferences. The way in which midwives portray information is also very influential. Therefore, probabilities should be presented in a number of ways and care should be taken to sequence information appropriately. When weighing up the options, there is a tendency to over-simplify information using rules of thumb and previous experiences. The midwife should identify misconceptions and aim to correct these before decisions are made.

The decision-making process requires clinical judgement and a degree of flexibility, but there are certain practice principles that apply. First, the presumption should be that women wish to be well informed and included in care planning. Second, information should be based on the best current evidence and should be presented in a balanced way. Third, written information is a useful supplement to face-to-face discussion, but it is not a substitute. Finally, midwives should respect the fact that women may not share their views when deciding how to proceed. These principles enable trusting professional relationships to develop. In short, involving parents in decision making is at the core of midwifery practice.

References

1. Perceval JT. Extract from: A narrative of the treatment received by a gentleman during a state of mental derangement (first published in 1838–1840). In: Porter R. The Faber book of madness. London: Faber and Faber; 1991:246–247.

2. Nursing and Midwifery Council. Midwives' rules and standards. London: NMC; 2004.

3. Department of Health. Building on the best: choice, responsiveness and equity in the NHS. London: The Stationery Office (TSO); 2003.

4. Norain J, Finney S. Parents of Down's girl are in line for £500 000. Daily Mail: Saturday May 17; 2003:29.

5. Marteau TM, Dormandy E, Michie S. A measure of informed choice. Health Expectations 2001; 4:99–108.

6. Sullivan A. Skilled decision making: the blood supply of midwifery practice. In: Raynor M, Marshall J, Sullivan A eds. Decision making in midwifery practice. Oxford: Elsevier; 2005:175–182.

7. Briss P, Rimer B, Reilly B, et al. Promoting informed choices about cancer screening in communities and healthcare systems. American Journal of Preventive Medicine 2004; 26(1):67–80.

8. Heyman B, Henrikson M, Maughan K. Probabilities and health risks: a qualitative approach. Social Science and Medicine 1998; 47(9):1295–1306.

9. Department of Health. Good practice in consent implementation guide: consent to examination or treatment. London: Department of Health. Crown Copyright; 2001.

10. Green JM, Hewison J, Bekker HL, et al. Psychosocial aspects of genetic screening of pregnant women and newborns: a systematic review. Health Technology Assessment 2004; 8(33):30.

11. Shrauger JS, Mariano E, Wlater TJ. Depressive symptoms and accuracy in the prediction of future events. Personality and Social Psychology Bulletin 1998; 24(8):880–892.

3

Pregnancy loss, breaking bad news and supporting parents

Jane Fisher

THE IMPACT OF PREGNANCY LOSS

Once a pregnancy is confirmed, women and their partners will bring with them to any consultation with a health professional a wide variety of emotions and expectations, which may include excitement and joy on the one hand and perhaps fear and trepidation on the other. Some may have ambivalent feelings about the pregnancy. In some cases, feelings change as the pregnancy progresses.

The plethora of meanings a particular parent or couple ascribes to a pregnancy will mean that news that it is not viable, that the baby has miscarried, died or has an abnormality will have an impact which will vary in its intensity. We know that the health professionals involved at this time cannot take away the pain and distress this causes, but research has shown that sensitive management of care that takes into account parents' feelings can help ensure that this distress is not exacerbated and that parents can take away some positive memories from such a difficult experience. A midwife is in the position of being able to develop a relationship with the parents that can help ensure that they receive the necessary compassion, continuity and consistency of care to help them through the loss and its aftermath.

Whatever the nature or timing of the pregnancy loss, there should never be assumptions made about its meaning for the parents involved or the impact it has. While some professionals may have years of experience of dealing with pregnancy loss and have built up their own ideas of its significance for parents, an individual loss is just that—a very individual experience for the woman or couple. It is dangerous to assume that an early miscarriage will always be easier to bear than an intrauterine death in the second trimester. However, this chapter will explore in some detail the circumstances surrounding a termination of pregnancy after the diagnosis of abnormality, not because it is a more significant loss, but because there may be specific considerations for health professionals when supporting parents during and after the decision-making process that is involved.

Dealing with parents in distress places great demands on their healthcare practitioners.[1] On a professional level, it requires highly developed communication and support skills. On a personal level, it can touch on and arouse individual feelings of sadness and loss. This chapter can only go some way to presenting guidelines for best practice in this area, as it is essential that this is underpinned by the provision of appropriate training and structured support.

What follows is informed by research into pregnancy loss and the psychosocial sequelae[2–5] and by feedback given to the organisation Antenatal Results and Choices (ARC) by parents.

I'm sorry to have to tell you...

Bad news in pregnancy can come at any stage from the early indications of a non-viable pregnancy, miscarriage, intrauterine death, through to serious abnormality detected at an ultrasound scan or diagnosis of chromosomal abnormality from invasive testing. Whenever it occurs the impact cannot be underestimated. As this quote underlines, there is little solace for this woman that the news came at her 12-week rather than 20 week scan: '. . . then he said that I was lucky that the abnormality was found at 12 weeks and not later. But I did not think myself lucky at all.' (ARC News March 2000; diagnosis of anencephaly.)

It is important not to overlook the fact that news that their baby has a condition that health professionals would consider as 'minor' or treatable is still significant for parents and its impact should be acknowledged.[6] Parents will have to deal with the shock that the baby is 'different' from the fantasy they had built their expectations around. While most will come to an acceptance of this, they may need time to do so and support around and acknowledgement of their feelings.

Reporting screening results

With the introduction of universal screening for Down's syndrome,[7] all women are faced with the choice of whether or not to have a screening test. Most women enter the screening process expecting reassurance, but for a significant minority of women whose results prompt the offer of an invasive test, this will feel very much like 'bad news' about the pregnancy and will evoke shock and anxiety.

The way the result is reported can go some way towards enabling a woman to make sense of it in a way that will help her decide on the next steps. There is likely to be raised anxiety if her result means that she is offered an invasive test and this will require sensitive management by a midwife. For many women, being told that their screening test result has come back 'high risk' or 'at increased risk' can be unhelpful. These emotive phrases colour their interpretation of the statistic and can make it extremely difficult to view it realistically or in a way that is meaningful to the individual woman. This is particularly true for those women who are given a result described as 'high risk' or at increased risk between 1:100 and 1:200 and then find out that a similar statistic is used to describe the 'small' risk of miscarriage associated with invasive procedures.

While it is crucial that false reassurance is not given, women may need help making sense of their result in their own way. A variety of approaches can be useful, including visual representations of the result, or reframing it as a percentage, e.g. 1:100 could be expressed as a 1% chance that the baby has Down's syndrome or a 99% chance that it does not.[8] This is discussed in more detail in Chapter 2.

Whether or not a woman opts to have a diagnostic test, residual anxiety could remain with her for the rest of the pregnancy and she may wish to talk her worries through with her midwife. The wait for a result from chorionic villus sampling (CVS) or amniocentesis can be a particularly anxious time and we should not assume that all the anxieties disappear when a test result rules out Down's syndrome.[9]

BREAKING BAD NEWS

Although women and their partners will have individual needs which should be recognised and respected, there are general principles which can be applied to breaking bad news.

Find the most appropriate place available

In a busy hospital setting, it can be a challenge to find a quiet, private space to break bad news, although every effort should be made to do so. If it does prove impossible to find a private room, then the health professional should acknowledge the less than ideal setting and make every effort to create a 'safe space', where parents feel they matter. This could include arranging chairs facing each other, minimising possible distractions (taking phones off the hook, turning off mobiles, etc.) and alerting other staff to help avoid interruptions.

When the setting is the scan room, there are no options as to where disclosure takes place, though there may be considerations such as does the woman want to get dressed and sit up to talk? Or would she rather be shown the findings on scan first?

Express sympathy and concern

'I'm sorry to have to tell you . . .' 'I'm afraid I have some bad news.' 'I'm so sorry, this must come as a terrible shock.' 'I can see this is difficult for you.'

Parents appreciate acknowledgement of the sadness of the situation; empathy from a health professional allows/enables parents to express their own feelings and the meaning the news has for them. In this difficult and sometimes overwhelm-

ing process it can help parents know that they and their feelings matter.

Be clear, honest and open

It is crucial that parents are provided with clear information, and that the seriousness of any finding is not played down as this could provide false reassurance. The information should be as full as is possible, but initially there may be limits to the amount of information a health professional has and can give. It is important to be honest about the extent of your knowledge and parents need to know how and when further information will be provided. If the problem has been found on scan, it may need to be confirmed by a consultant, or further scanning may be required. If it is an unusual karyotype a later appointment with a specialist genetic counsellor may be needed. These difficulties are often unavoidable, but the wait for follow-up should be minimal and the anxiety involved acknowledged

Give time

News of an abnormality or of the death in utero of a baby is going to come as a shock to parents—even if they have come to a consultation knowing there is cause for concern. Shock manifests itself in different ways, but for most people it means that assimilating information will be hard. This means information has to be paced carefully. It is best to take a cue from the parents—what is their body language communicating? Are they unable to make eye contact or have they 'closed down'? It can be useful to say something like: 'I realise this is upsetting for you—please stop me if you've heard enough or it gets too much to take in.'

Couples may need to be left on their own after part of the consultation in order to give each other emotional support or try to make sense of what they have been told in their own time.

Categorise information

To aid understanding, explanations should follow a logical sequence. A possible strategy is to say: 'I am going to go through what I have found on the scan/what has been diagnosed by the test, we can then talk about what it might mean for your baby and what the next steps are. Please stop me at any time if something is unclear or if you have any questions.'

Do not overload with information

Because of the difficulties with assimilation, there may be a limit to what the parents can take in. If they need to go away with vital information it will help if they can leave with something written to consolidate what has been said. If it is proving impossible to communicate effectively it will be necessary to offer another appointment.

Use clear, jargon-free language

Parents need to have a clear understanding of what has been found in their baby and its implications. It is not helpful if health professionals are euphemistic in their use of language or offer parents false hope because of a desire to protect them from the 'harsh' truth.

If a parent is told at an early scan, when the professional involved knows that the baby is dead, 'I'm afraid I can't find your baby's heartbeat' then that parent may be justified in responding with 'Well, if you can't find it, find me someone who can!' There will be no such misunderstanding if the parent is told: 'I'm afraid there is no heartbeat, which sadly means your baby has died—I'm very sorry.'

There is widespread use of jargon in all professions, but for those outside a profession it can be impossible to understand, so it should be avoided when speaking to parents. There will be times when medical terminology will have to be used, and it is important that parents know the correct terminology and have it explained to them.

An example of this may be:

I'm sorry that I am going to give you some painful news. The amniocentesis results show us that your baby has Patau's syndrome. This is a serious chromosomal abnormality which is also known as trisomy 13, because the baby has three chromosome 13s in all its cells instead of the usual two. I'm afraid the implications for your baby are severe and very few babies with Patau's survive to birth. Those that do will die some time afterwards.

Check for understanding

Following the diagnosis of Down's syndrome from a CVS or amniocentesis, you may need to check what a parent knows about Down's syndrome. In order to obtain as complete an answer as possible and get some understanding of what the diagnosis might mean for the parent it will be necessary to gently question them. If asked, 'Do you know about Down's syndrome?' or 'Do you have an understanding of the condition?' a parent who answers 'yes' has given nothing away about their level of knowledge or what it means to them. A more open question will enable you to find out much more. 'Can you tell me a bit about what you know about Down's syndrome, so I can perhaps help you fill in any gaps?' In other circumstances a useful way of checking understanding is to gently ask, 'Can I just ask you to tell me what you've understood of what I've told you so that I can be sure that I have explained it properly?'

In some cases parents may have acquired their own knowledge about a condition, perhaps from family, friends or the media, which is factually incorrect. It can be difficult to contradict them if they have chosen to be very positive about the outlook and you know that the reality is different. However, it is clearly important that they have as accurate a picture of the prognosis as possible. It may be useful to fix appointments with other health professionals who you know to be familiar with the condition and perhaps provide written information or recommend relevant support groups or useful internet sites.

When dealing with parents who do not speak English, the services of a briefed and trusted interpreter are essential. If the only option is to ask a relative or friend to translate, every attempt should be made to check that they have a good understanding of the situation and that their approach is non-directive.

There can be difficulties when a miscarriage is confirmed when there is no definitive explanation for the spontaneous loss, or when the reason for it can be attributed to something the woman has or has not done. In such circumstances, the woman may experience a range of emotions and the provision of ongoing support may be required.

Be prepared for a range of responses

People react to shock in many different ways. Reactions can range from anger, denial and high emotion to acceptance or impenetrable silence. Depending on a professional's personal and cultural experience, some responses will be more difficult to cope with than others. Reflecting on the most demanding scenarios and sharing these with colleagues can increase confidence.

Extreme anger can be particularly difficult and sometimes frightening. No professional should be made to feel at risk of injury and it may be that a statement such as: 'I appreciate that you're angry, but your behaviour is making me feel threatened and so I'm going to have to call a colleague' can be enough to dissipate the threat.

A reaction of calm acceptance should not preclude careful checking of understanding and an offer of support.

What happens next?

As the consultation draws to a close, there will be a number of factors to consider before the parent leaves you and it may be useful to have the following questions to hand:

- Do the parents have to wait to see someone else—if so where will they wait? If a woman is alone, is there someone who can stay with her? Can the parents avoid being faced with other expectant mothers?
- Is there a member of staff who can be with them and offer immediate support when they leave you?
- Are they clear on the next steps—do they have written information about the next appointment?
- Is there someone they can contact before that appointment if they have concerns?
- Have they got contact details of any relevant support groups?
- Are the parents too distressed to drive home safely? Is there someone who can come and collect them in this instance?

It may be appropriate to end the consultation by reiterating how sorry you are about their baby—a physical gesture such as a touch on the arm can emphasise this sympathy.

Support for the health professional

Depending on the setting and the timing of the consultation at which you have broken bad news, immediate support may not be available. However, it is crucial that health professionals involved in the delivery of distressing news to parents do have the chance to debrief and gain support.

Giving results over the phone

Although this is not ideal, sometimes bad news will be broken over the phone, e.g. the results of a CVS or amniocentesis. This can be especially challenging as a health professional cannot see parents' reactions and try to read their body language to help assess the impact the news has had. In these circumstances it will be particularly important to pace the information carefully, allowing silences and checking regularly for understanding. It will be necessary to listen effectively to what the parent does and does not say and their tone. A follow-up face-to-face appointment should be arranged as soon as possible and parents should be given a number to contact in the meantime if they have questions or want support.

SUPPORTING PARENTS AFTER A DIAGNOSIS OF ABNORMALITY

After the diagnosis of an abnormality, parents will have a variety of needs. They will be dealing with the shock that something is wrong with the baby they are carrying and often grieving for the 'healthy' baby they had formerly been building their hopes and dreams around.

If the condition affecting the baby has raised the possibility of termination for parents, they have to embark on a painful decision-making process at a time when they perhaps feel least equipped to cope with the emotional demands this will put upon them. It is paramount that in these circumstances parents have access to all the relevant information and support available so that they can make a decision which is appropriate to their individual situation. Those caring for them have a responsibility to offer help to enable them to make the choice that they will best be able to live with.

Parents have often reported that the parent handbooks produced by ARC[10,11] can be particularly useful, as they clearly and sensitively outline the issues and options that may be encountered by parents on either journey.

The decision-making process

When parents have all the available information on the abnormality diagnosed in their baby, they will need care and support during the process of decision making. Some will need more than others. It can be helpful if they have a designated health professional who can act as a key worker and maintain continuity and consistency. This person should be easy to contact and should help set up further consultations with doctors if required, and signpost parents to other sources of information and support.

In order to come to a decision, parents will need clear, consistent information about the condition affecting their baby. In certain circumstances, there may only be limited information available, or there may be great uncertainty about the prognosis. Parents' anxiety in this situation should be acknowledged.

The information parents may want is shown in Box 3.1.

Sometimes parents will need to be directed to more than one source to gather information; this is where having a midwife's help can be invaluable in providing a consistent point during these referrals. Where possible it will be beneficial for a midwife to sit in during consultations so as to keep a record of what has been said and to help make sure that all the parents' concerns are covered.

Parents will want to feel that they have had adequate time to come to a decision and have not been 'railroaded' or rushed. There will be those who come to a decision quite swiftly, others may need longer. There may be practical difficulties about this if, for example, the baby's gestation is approaching 24 weeks, as there is greater limitation on accessing terminations after this. Parents appreciate being told if and why there are time con-

Box 3.1   Information to help parents come to a decision

- A clear explanation of the anomaly
- The certainty of the diagnosis. If it is not certain, how and when it will be confirmed and whether they will be referred to a specialist unit
- How the pregnancy is likely to progress
- Whether special care or treatment will be required before birth
- What the longer-term prognosis is for the baby and what treatment might be available
- How the condition will affect their child's quality of life
- Sources of more information about living with the condition
- What will happen if they decide to continue or end the pregnancy.

straints on their decision making. If there are constraints, the quality of the consultations is extremely important and it can be useful to refer parents to other organisations for support, i.e. the ARC helpline (see end of chapter).

There may be those who feel they have considered the options from every angle and become distressed at the difficulty they experience in coming to a final decision—the feeling that they are tortuously 'going round in circles'. They can be reassured that this vacillation is a normal part of the decision-making process.

Parents benefit from contact with healthcare professionals who are responsive to their individual needs. Those caring for them need to have or develop the necessary skills to be able to help explore the possible outcomes and parents' feelings about them. Listening skills are particularly important in order to understand what the situation means for parents and what their individual needs are. Some parents will need someone who can help them to articulate what can be very painful emotions and then to accept the decision they have made but find it difficult to come to terms with. It will aid their emotional recovery if they can look back and believe that they made the best decision they could in the circumstances. There is currently much emphasis on health professionals taking a non-directive approach and while all will agree that parents have to make their own decision, they can sometimes feel very alone in facing what seems an impossible task. This is a very delicate and difficult area for practitioners as they need to provide the help and support that will prevent parents from feeling 'abandoned'.

Sometimes parents may ask questions such as 'What would you do?' or 'What should I do?' Because of the desire to be non-directive, the temptation can be to evade or gloss over such questions. It is more helpful for parents if the difficulty of their situation and the anxiety raised by dilemmas they face is acknowledged. Though no health professional can make decisions for parents, they can support them and help provide a framework to guide them to the choice that is appropriate to their individual circumstances. More guidance on effectively supporting decision making is given in an ARC booklet for professionals.[12]

Professional attitudes and beliefs

The worst thing I find is not being able to tell just anyone for fear of them not understanding or even being vehemently against me—normally I can argue my corner well but I still feel too emotionally bruised to defend my decision. People with newborn babies still avoid me for fear of hurting me. They don't realise that they hurt me more by staying away or by not offering me their baby to hold or by generally avoiding the subject of babies. This has at times left me feeling isolated in my feelings and unable to give them an outlet.

(ARC News March 2001; mother who had a termination after a diagnosis of Down's syndrome.)

The majority of midwives come into the profession with a desire to be part of a joyous time in family life; and most of the time this ambition will be fulfilled. However, more than a fifth of parents will experience a miscarriage and 2% will be told their baby has a serious abnormality. Some of the latter will consider the possibility of termination. Just as in the general population, there will be midwives who have strong feelings about when or if termination is ever justified. We all have and are entitled to our personal attitudes and beliefs, but we also have a duty to recognise when these attitudes may impede our ability to

provide best care for others. It is obviously essential that parents are not met with 'disapproval' for a course of action they are taking or considering. When coming to a decision parents are sometimes especially sensitive to the reactions and attitudes of others.

Continuity of care

Everyone was extremely kind and supportive, but the communication between them was appalling and I constantly had to explain what was happening to me and why I was there.

(ARC News March 2000; woman whose baby was diagnosed with a heart defect.)

In the case of pregnancy loss or the diagnosis of abnormality, there needs to be a multidisciplinary approach so that all health professionals the parents may come into contact with are conversant with their situation. There can be added distress if different health professionals are not consistent in the information they give. To avoid problems, it can be helpful to the parents to have a midwife who acts as a 'key professional' for them. It should be someone who the parents can contact easily and who is able to signpost them to accessing what they need. According to the way antenatal care is structured, it may be necessary that all those in a team involved with the parents have good liaison to maintain this continuity.

SUPPORT AFTER A BEREAVEMENT

Remembering the baby

Depending on the circumstances of the loss, there may be a number of choices for parents to consider in relation to remembering their baby. Although it can seem (sometimes to parents themselves) that thinking about funeral arrangements or whether to see and hold the baby is adding layers of distress, it is important for parents to be involved in decision making at a time when they can think that everything is outside their control. Not knowing that certain options were open to them at the time and only learning of them later can indeed add to their distress.

There are no right and wrong ways about how parents choose to handle what happens after the death of a baby. Though it is true that parents rarely regret seeing and spending time with their dead baby, many choose not to do so knowing it is the right decision for them. Some name their baby and are keen to know the sex, others always refer to a fetus and entrust all arrangements to the hospital. Parents need to know what is available and be reassured that they do not always have to make immediate hard and fast decisions. They can see their baby later rather than sooner. Sometimes they can be given the confidence to do this by a midwife talking beforehand about how the baby is likely to look and then after the birth describing the baby to them.

Some parents want their baby dressed in clothes they have bought; some want to help bath the baby; others may want to take their baby home. As far as possible, all requests should be accommodated and a clear explanation given if a wish cannot be granted.

Babies who die after 24 weeks' gestation are automatically registered as a stillbirth, but some parents want written acknowledgement of a baby who died earlier. In this circumstance hospitals could offer their own certification, or at least should enable parents to write in a book of remembrance.

Details of the legal requirements for registration and guidelines for procedures before 24 weeks can be found at this Department of Health site page: http://www.dh.gov.uk/PolicyAndGuidance/Health AndSocialCareTopics/Tissue/TissueGeneralInforma tion/fs/en.

For those parents who have an early first trimester miscarriage,[14] there may be nothing tangible, such as a scan picture, which can act as a keepsake. If they are encouraged to explore their feelings and the meaning the loss represents for them, strategies can be discussed to help them acknowledge the loss in a way they feel comfortable with.

Parents value above all else being treated with respect and having that same respect afforded to their baby.

Post mortems

We decided to allow a post mortem in case it was a genetic problem. I couldn't stop thinking about her. I didn't want to leave her. I wanted to make sure she

was being loved. I know she was dead but she was still my baby and I loved her—dead or alive. I didn't sleep properly over the nights. I knew she was being transported around to different places. Just as if you had a live baby you wouldn't leave it alone. I didn't want to do this with my dead baby but obviously I had no choice—did this get any easier? Were these people being careful with my baby? I called the hospital one day to see if she had arrived back from the post mortem. The man said that the van arrives later with the load. I was so hurt and then to hear a strange man say my baby was part of a load just topped it off really. When I knew she was back at the hospital I felt better.'

(ARC News July 2001; woman who had a termination after a diagnosis of atrial septal defect.)

Although discussions around post mortem may be had with one health professional, parents may often want to discuss their feelings and final decision with someone else they trust. If midwives are involved in discussions with parents it will be important for them to check if parents are aware of the information a post-mortem report could provide and its significance for future pregnancies.

Funerals and disposal

If you ask me four years later what was the worst part of the whole ordeal, my answer would be leaving him. I quite literally could have put him in my case and walked away with him. It tormented me so much that the following afternoon I returned to the hospital to be with him again. The same compassion was shown, the midwives were still there to support me, and took the opportunity to talk to me about the funeral... I said my last goodbye to him that Monday afternoon. That was the last time I saw him, touched him and kissed him.

(ARC News October 2002; woman who had termination after a diagnosis of anencephaly.)

The options around funeral or disposal arrangements should be made explicit to parents. They need to know what the hospital offers and what they can access privately. If parents want a cremation, they might need to be prepared for the fact that there may not be ashes available to them.

Those whose baby dies before 24 weeks and who want the hospital to deal with the remains, may come back in the future with questions about what happened. It is therefore useful if staff know what hospital procedures are and these procedures ensure that the remains are treated with dignity.

Partners

When our world fell apart, I subconsciously assumed the 'strong' role—dealing with the outside world, showing a brave face, but in retrospect not realising that by hiding my own grief I was giving the impression of being uncaring. This may not ring true for all men, but I bet it does for quite a few.

I did not want to arrive at the hospital; I did not want to sit in the waiting room; I did not want to hear my wife's footsteps coming into the waiting room and I did not want to hear the consultant call my wife to the room to stop my son's heart. But I did. As soon as I said my farewells to my son as I sat outside the room, I suddenly felt calm—I felt a warm feeling come down my neck and over my shoulders. He had touched me as he had gone. And almost immediately the midwife called me into the room—my wife in tears, my son was dead. It was a time of profound grief. The midwife and consultant treated us with respect and care. They were fabulous.

(ARC News July 2003; father describing feticide.)

It is often the case that care in the context of pregnancy loss is concentrated on the mother. Partners will say themselves that they neglect their own needs in favour of taking on a supportive or practical role. It is vital to remember that partners have had a significant loss too and will have their own feelings and needs that are always in danger of being subsumed in those of the mother. An added burden for many is watching the mother suffer and having no power to take any of the pain or distress away. For men who have been brought up not to show their feelings, articulating their own pain and needs can be hard.

There is sometimes an added complication if the couple feel differently about how to proceed. In the case of a diagnosis of abnormality it could be that one partner feels differently about the future of the pregnancy. If the couple are unable to come to agreement there may be the need for a third party, perhaps a counselling midwife, to intervene.

Follow-up care

Everything went smoothly, but it was afterwards I felt so lonely. I had no visits from doctors, health visitors or midwives and now, 17 months on I am on a course of tablets for depression. It took me a good 12 months to finally visit the doctor and tell him my feelings. I felt as if nobody wanted to talk about my baby and my experiences and feelings, and because I had three other children I should just get on with my life and forget about the past. I couldn't do that, just because I have children to keep me busy it never stops me thinking about the daughter I lost.

(ARC News October 2002; woman who had termination after a diagnosis of spina bifida.)

Research suggests that parents appreciate the provision of ongoing care in the period after their bereavement. They will vary in the nature and amount of care they want. If help is offered parents can refuse and many will appreciate a visit from a midwife they had a good relationship with. As well as raising any concerns about their physical recovery, such a visit will give women (and their partners) the opportunity to talk about their experience.

Again, it is crucial that those involved in primary care are fully informed, so that health visitors or GPs do not contact bereaved parents assuming the birth of a live baby.

The pregnancy after a loss

I'd say it took me almost a year to feel normal again. I thought my heart would break and I was desperate for another baby to replace the one I'd lost, which of course could never be done. I knew I had the support of friends and family, and especially from the specialist midwife who later became a great friend, but although I wanted to, I couldn't talk about it, it was too painful. I felt like a failure and although rationally I knew it was unlikely to happen again, I was very frightened that it would.

(ARC News December 2004; woman whose baby had Edward's syndrome.)

For parents, deciding to become pregnant again after a loss can be a source of great hope. Some desperately want to have another baby and become distressed when it does not happen as soon as they would like. Others struggle over deciding whether and when to try to conceive again, and this in itself can be emotionally painful.

When a couple do successfully conceive again, the initial joy is often clouded by conflicting feelings. They may feel guilt at trying to 'replace' or fear of forgetting the baby that died. They may worry about the same thing happening again. They will have questions about management of this pregnancy that they might appreciate talking over with their previous midwife. If they were happy with the care last time round they may want to be under the same practitioners' care. If they have particularly bad memories they may want to avoid certain personnel or even book with a different unit.

Care should be taken that parents have access to all the screening and diagnostic tests they want, as early as possible, where practicable and that they have all the support they need. The point in the pregnancy where the previous loss was experienced or abnormality was first detected can be particularly stressful. There may well be anxiety until the baby actually arrives, even if the indicators are positive throughout. Even the joy in the aftermath of birth may be mixed with painful emotions related to their previous experience.

It can help parents if all the staff they meet are aware of their history and sensitive to the implications this may have. Some will want to be scanned by the same sonographer who detected problems last time, as he or she was one of the few who were privy to their baby's brief existence. For others this may be something they are anxious to avoid. Gentle probing and ongoing support from a midwife can enable parents to express their preferences.

STAFF TRAINING AND SUPPORT

Working with women and couples who are distressed or bereaved is demanding and will draw heavily on personal resources. In order to ensure that they can give good care consistently, it is essential that staff have recourse to structured support and ongoing training. Only when such provision is in place will staff be equipped with the emotional capacity and requisite skills to provide a gold standard of care to parents at a poignant and sensitive time in their lives.

Key Practice Points

- Whatever the nature or timing of the pregnancy loss, there should never be assumptions made about its meaning for the parents involved or the impact it has.
- Find the most appropriate and suitable place available when breaking bad news.
- Express sympathy and concern.
- Be clear honest and open.
- Give time.
- Categorise information but do not overload.
- Use clear jargon-free language and check parents' understanding.
- Be prepared for a range of responses.

References

1. Kohner N. Pregnancy loss and the death of a baby: guidelines for professionals. 2nd edn. SANDS London 1996.
2. Statham H, Solomou W, et al. Prenatal diagnosis of fetal abnormality: psychological effects on women in low-risk pregnancies. Baillière's Clinical Obstetrics and Gynaecology 2000; 14(4):731–747.
3. Statham H. Prenatal diagnosis of fetal abnormality: the decision to terminate the pregnancy and the psychological consequences. Fetal and Maternal Medicine Review 2002; 13:213–247.
4. Lasker JN, Toedter LJ. Predicting outcomes after pregnancy loss; results from studies using the Perinatal Grief Scale. Illness, Crisis and Loss 2000; 8(4):350–372.
5. Toedter LJ, Lasker JN, et al. International comparison of studies using the Perinatal Grief Scale: a decade of research on pregnancy loss. Death Studies 2001; 25:205–228.
6. Statham H, Solomou W, et al. Continuing a pregnancy after the diagnosis of an anomaly: parents' experiences. In: Abramsky L, Chapple J. Prenatal diagnosis: the human side. London: Chapman and Hall; 2003.
7. Department of Health Chief Executive Bulletin – 14 – 20 September 2001 Issue 84 NHS Interest (4)
8. Gates EA. Communicating risk in prenatal genetic testing. Journal of Midwifery and Women's Health 2004; 49:220–227.
9. Marteau TM, Mansfield CD. (1998). The psychological impact of prenatal diagnosis and subse-

quent decisions. Yearbook of Obstetrics and Gynaecology. P. M. S. O'Brien. London: RCOG; 1998:186–193.

10. ARC (Antenatal Results and Choices). A handbook to be given to parents when an abnormality is diagnosed in their unborn baby. 3rd edn. London: ARC; 1999.

11. ARC. Supporting you throughout your pregnancy: a handbook for parents after a prenatal diagnosis. London: ARC; 2003.

12. ARC. Supporting parents' decisions: a handbook for professionals. London: ARC; 2005.

13. Statham H, Solomou W, et al. Communication of prenatal screening and diagnosis results to primary-care health professionals. Public Health 2003; 117(5):348–357.

14. Thornstensen KA. Midwifery management of first trimester bleeding and early pregnancy loss. Journal of Midwifery and Women's Health 2000 Nov–Dec; 45(6):481–497.

Quotations in the text are from the ARC Members' Newsletter, ARC News, provided free to members of ARC three times a year.

UK Support Organisations

ARC Antenatal Results and Choices
Tel:0207 631 0280
www.arc-uk.org

Miscarriage Association
Tel:01924 200 799
www.miscarriage.association.org.uk

SANDS Stillbirth and Neonatal Death Society
Tel:0207 436 5881
www.uk-sands.org

Section Two

Maternal investigations

SECTION CONTENTS

Haematology in pregnancy

Jane Strong

INTRODUCTION

The aims of this chapter are to review the screening and management of problems grouped under the following major headings:

- Full blood count
- Haemoglobinopathy screens
- Thrombophilia and coagulation screens
- Red cell antibodies.

FULL BLOOD COUNT (FBC)[1]

This is the most frequently requested haematological test. Blood is taken into a bottle containing ethylene diamine tetra-acetic acid (EDTA), an anticoagulant, and processed through an automatic analyser. The results provide information on red cells, white cells and platelets.

Red cells

- Red cell count (RCC), i.e. the number of red cells
- Haematocrit (Hct)—the proportion of red cells in a column of centrifuged blood expressed as a decimal fraction.
- Haemoglobin (Hb)—the concentration of this specialised protein involved in carrying oxygen to the tissues and carbon dioxide from the tissue to the lungs.

From the above three measurements the size and haemoglobin content of the red cells can also be derived:

- Mean corpuscular volume (MCV)—gives information about the mean size of the red cells.

- Mean corpuscular haemoglobin (MCH)—indicates the mean amount of haemoglobin in the red cells.
- Mean corpuscular haemoglobin concentration (MCHC)—indicates the mean concentration of haemoglobin in a red cell (see Table 4.1).

White cells

The number of white cells is counted and different types of white cells are identified. This is known as a white cell differential. There are 5 different white cell types: neutrophils, lymphocytes, monocytes, eosinophils and basophils (see Table 4.2).

Table 4.1 **Red cell parameters in the full blood count (FBC)**

Parameter	Non-pregnant female	Pregnant woman	Diagnostic inference
Red cell count ($\times 10^{12}$/l)	4.0–5.2	Falls 3.1–4.4	↑ Polycythaemia ↓ Anaemia
Haemoglobin (g/dl)	12–15	Falls >11 1st & 3rd trimester, >10.5 2nd trimester	
Packed cell volume (PCV) or haematocrit (hct)	38–48% (also expressed as 0.38–0.48)	Falls 28–41%	
Mean cell volume (MCV) (fl)	80–100	Rises—on average 4–6 fl but rise of 20 fl reported	↑Macrocytic: ↑Reticulocytes Liver disease Hypothyroidism ↓B12 ↓Folate ↓ Microcytic: Iron deficiency Thalassaemia Anaemia of chronic disease
Mean cell haemoglobin (MCH)(pg)	27–32		↓Hypochromia
Mean cell haemoglobin concentration (MCHC)(g/dl)	32–36		Occurs with microcytosis
Reticulocyte count	1–2% circulating red blood cells 10–100 $\times 10^9$/l	↑ with peak levels of 6% at 25–30 weeks	↑Reticulocytosis: Haemolysis after acute blood loss ↓Reticulocytopenia: Impaired red cell production

Table 4.2 **White cell and platelet parameters in the full blood count (FBC)**

Parameter	Normal non-pregnant range	Changes in pregnancy	Classification—values outside the normal range	Diagnostic inference
White cell count (WCC) ($\times 10^9$/l)	4–11	Rise: Left shift occurs 5.7–16.9	↑leucocytosis ↓leucopaenia	Dependent on the part of the WCC that is low— see below
Neutrophils ($\times 10^9$/l)	2–7.5 (40–80%)	Rise 3.6–13.1	↑neutrophilia	Infection Inflammation Acute haemorrhage Steroids Smoking Pre-eclampsia Myeloproliferative Leukaemic disorders
			↓neutropaenia	Immune Infection Drugs Part of pancytopenia
Lymphocytes ($\times 10^9$/l)	1.2–4.0 (20–40%)	Fall 0.9–3.9	↑lymphocytosis	Viral infections Some bacterial infections Smoking Splenectomy
			↓lymphopaenia	Acute stress Steroids Autoimmune conditions End stage HIV
Monocytes ($\times 10^9$/l)	0.2–0.8 (2–10%)	Rise 0.3–1.1	↑monocytosis	Chronic infection or inflammation
Eosinophils ($\times 10^9$/l)	0.04–0.44 (1–6%)	Fall 0–0.33	↑eosinophilia	Allergic diseases Drug hypersensitivity Parasitic infections Skin diseases
Basophils ($\times 10^9$/l)	0–0.1 (<1–2%)	Fall 0.0–0.09	↑basophilia	Reactive Myeloproliferative and leukaemic disorders
Platelets $\times 10^9$/l	150–400	10% decline over non-pregnant values—same normal range quoted i.e. 150–400	↑thrombocytosis	Reactive to haemorrhage, infection, inflammation, malignancy Primary—essential thrombocythaemia: primary bone marrow disorder, myeloproliferative condition

table continues

Table 4.2   White cell and platelet parameters in the full blood count (FBC)—Cont'd

Parameter	Normal non-pregnant range	Changes in pregnancy	Classification— values outside the normal range	Diagnostic inference
			↓thrombocytopenia	Gestational or incidental thrombocytopenia of pregnancy Hypertensive disorders of pregnancy Immune thrombo- cytopenia Primary bone marrow disorders

Platelets

The number of platelets is counted and their size is sometimes available expressed as a mean platelet volume (MPV) (see Table 4.2).

Physiological changes in pregnancy[2]

Red cells

The number of red cells increases in pregnancy by 18–25%, but the volume of plasma increases to a greater extent—by 40–50%. This results in a decreased haematocrit and a dilutional drop in haemoglobin. This starts at 10 weeks of gestation, is maximal at 32–34 weeks and recovers by 5–7 days after delivery. The expanded blood volume meets the demands of the uteroplacental unit, and protects against impaired venous return and also blood loss at delivery. Normal haemoglobin values in pregnancy should be at least 11 g/dl in the first and third trimesters and above 10.5 g/dl in the second trimester.

There is a small physiological increase in mean corpuscular volume (MCV)—on average 4–6 fl but the increase may be as much as 20 fl. MCH and MCHC are unchanged in pregnancy (see Table 4.1).

White cells

The total white cell count rises throughout pregnancy and these changes are often still present 6–8 weeks post delivery. Minimal changes occur in the numbers of circulating lymphocytes and mono-cytes. Eosinophils fall in the third trimester. Neutrophils rise throughout pregnancy and it is not unusual to see immature neutrophils (myelo-cytes and metamyelocytes) in peripheral blood films in pregnancy. This is known as a left shift in the white cell differential (see Table 4.1).

Platelets

Maternal platelet counts fall during pregnancy. This is most marked in the third trimester. About 5% of pregnancies will have a platelet count lower than 150×10^9/l that is physiological and without consequence for either mother or fetus. It is the most common reason for a low platelet count in pregnancy and generally resolves within 6 weeks of delivery. The platelet count is usually above 100×10^9/l and rarely below 70×10^9/l in this incidental thrombocytopenia of pregnancy. The most useful indicators that the platelet drop is physiological include the timing of the platelet count drop, the platelet count level, and resolution after delivery, normal cord platelet count and the knowledge that the platelet count was normal pre pregnancy (see Table 4.1).

Rationales for investigations

The National Institute for Clinical Excellence (NICE) antenatal care guideline[3] recommends that an FBC should be tested at booking and at 28 weeks and this should be repeated at least once in the postpartum period. This is primarily to screen for anaemia. If there are abnormalities more frequent monitoring is appropriate. The frequency of FBC testing depends on the abnormality and the treatment given.

General guidance when interpreting the FBC

Remember normal ranges quoted on full blood count reports are not for the pregnant population—they relate to an adult population. The physiological changes that occur in pregnancy need to be kept in mind when interpreting a pregnant woman's full blood count.

When interpreting FBC results have a systematic approach:

- Is the haemoglobin normal? If not is it low or high? If low is there any clue from the size and haemoglobin content of the red cells as to why this may be? Are there any blood film comments that help?
- Then move onto the white cell count. Is it normal, high or low? Which part of the differential count is abnormal (i.e. neutrophils, lymphocytes, monocytes, eosinophils or basophils)? Are there any blood film comments that help?
- Then move onto the platelet count. Is it normal, low or high? Are there any comments on the blood film that help?

It is useful to think of an FBC as the products of a blood making factory—the bone marrow. The bone marrow is made up of different departments making the three products—red cells, white cells and platelets. How many departments of the bone marrow is the abnormality affecting? If more than one department is affected, conditions causing bone marrow failure should be considered in the differential diagnosis.

Reticulocytes

Reticulocytes are immature red cells newly released from the bone marrow. This test is not automatically performed as part of the FBC but can be analysed from the same ethylene diamine tetra acetic acid (EDTA) sample. It needs to be specifically requested. The sample needs to be fresh. Some automatic analysers are able to estimate the numbers of these cells. Alternatively, they are manually counted on a spe-

cially stained blood film. The normal reticulocyte count is 1–2%. This measurement can be useful in ascertaining whether a low haemoglobin is the result of decreased marrow red cell production or increased red cell destruction. The reticulocyte count will be low in the former and increased in the latter.

Blood film

This is made by placing a drop of blood near one end of a glass slide. A spreader is applied in front of the drop of blood and drawn back into it until the blood has spread along the back edge of the spreader, which is then advanced over the slide so a thin film of blood is spread over the slide. These wedge spread films can also be prepared by mechanical spreaders and stained as part of the automation of FBCs. Examination of the blood film allows the size, shape, appearance and number of all cell types to be evaluated (see Table 4.3).

Subsequent actions[4]

Anaemia—low haemoglobin for pregnancy (i.e. Hb<11 g/dl first and third trimesters, 10.5 g/dl second trimester)

Women with haemoglobins less than 9 g/dl should be referred for an obstetric haematology opinion. This should be a matter of urgency if in the third trimester. Referral is also required if there are white cell and or platelet abnormalities in addition to the anaemia.

The most common cause of anaemia in pregnancy is iron deficiency (over 90%). An effective diagnostic workup can therefore start with the question: does this patient have iron deficiency anaemia? Further workup will then depend on whether iron deficiency anaemia is confirmed or not.

Iron deficiency can be confirmed by a measure of iron stores. Ferritin is probably the most widely used estimate of iron stores. In iron deficiency anaemia ferritin levels are low. Ferritin is, however, an acute phase reactant and is an unreliable reflection of iron stores if there is active infection or inflammation.

The most common reason for iron deficiency anaemia in pregnancy is the increased demands of the fetus for iron. Demands are almost quadrupled from 2 mg/day initially up to 7 mg/day by term. For a pregnancy this equates to a total iron

Table 4.3   Red cell abnormalities on the blood film

Abnormality	Description	Diagnostic features
Microcytosis	Decrease in red cell size. Can be generalised or only affect a proportion of red cells. If generalised effect, the MCV will be reduced	See red cell parameters (Table 4.1)
Macrocytosis	Increase in red cell size—can be oval or round, and be general or only affect a proportion of red cells. If generalised effect, the MCV will be raised	See red cell parameters (Table 4.1)
Hypochromia	Reduced colour or staining of the red cell	Associated with microcytosis
Polychromasia (reticulocytosis)	Immature red cells with pinkish blue appearance, slighter larger than mature red cells	Increase and become noticeable in situations of increased red cell production such as blood loss or haemolysis
Poikilocytosis	Increased numbers of abnormally shaped red cells	
Spherocytosis	Spherical cells as opposed to the normal disciform	Hereditary spherocytosis, autoimmune haemolytic anaemia
Schistocytes	Fragments of red cells	Commonest cause is microangiopathic and mechanical haemolytic anaemia
Sickle cells	Red cells in the shape of a sickle	Sickling disorders
Target cells	Red cells with an increased area of staining centrally giving the appearance of a target	Liver disease, post splenectomy, haemoglobin C disease and trait

requirement of 800–1200 mg. Iron stores of at least 500 mg are required to withstand this demand without the development of iron deficiency. It is estimated that only 20% of menstruating women have stores of this magnitude. Risk factors for the development of iron deficiency in pregnancy include iron deficiency prior to pregnancy, hyperemesis, vegetarian or vegan diet, multiple pregnancies, pregnancy recurring after a short interval and blood loss.

Provided there are no unusual features to suggest another cause for the anaemia, treatment with iron can be started and a ferritin sent at the same time to confirm iron stores are low. The woman should be asked if she is known to have a haemoglobinopathy, whether she carries a haemoglobinopathy card or if she attends a haematology clinic for anaemia. These women should be referred directly to an obstetric haematology clinic for assessment.

Haemoglobin levels should rise 0.8 g/dl/week. Lack of clinical or haematological response after 3–4 weeks of oral iron therapy requires re-evaluation. In cases of failure to respond to oral iron, other causes for the anaemia should be considered, such as non-compliance, additional haematinic deficiencies, concomitant infections, or ongoing blood loss. These women should be referred for medical review (see Fig. 4.1).

Iron supplements tend to give gastrointestinal side effects dependent on the iron content. Dosage can be guided by the haemoglobin level. A suitable dose to begin with would be ferrous sulphate 200 mg once daily if the Hb is 9.5–10.5 g/dl in the third trimester or 9.5–11 g/dl on the booking sample. If the Hb is 8.0–9.4 the twice daily dosing is appropriate. Folate supplementation may also be helpful.

Polycythaemia—high haemoglobin >17 g/dl, haematocrit >0.56

Polycythaemia can be primary due to inappropriate marrow red cell production, or it can be secondary due to high erythropoietin levels. Levels may be

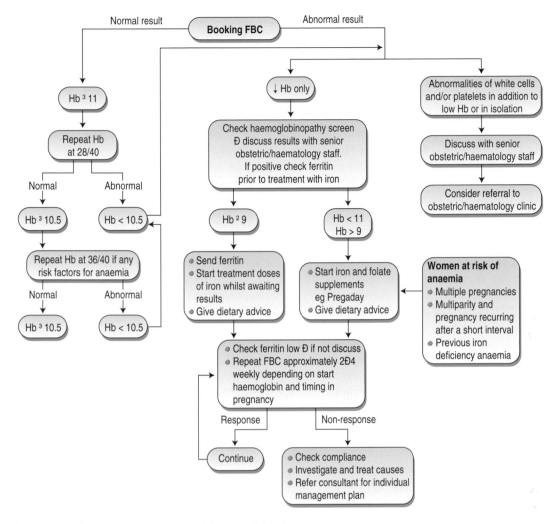

Figure 4.1 Management of antenatal haemoglobin levels.

appropriately elevated in the setting of tissue hypoxaemia or inappropriate overproduction by the liver, kidneys or tumours.

High haemoglobins are rare in pregnancy. In the first instance repeat the FBC. Ensure the woman is well hydrated.

Check for clinical symptoms associated with polycythaemia. These include headache, pruritis, weakness, dizziness and visual changes. Clinical signs include hypertension, gout and hepatosplenomegaly.

If the raised haemoglobin is confirmed, check oxygen saturation, uric acid, renal and liver func-

tion. Abdominal ultrasound of liver and kidneys is useful as is a chest X-ray and pulmonary function tests.

Outside of pregnancy the diagnostic test is the red cell mass study but this involves the use of radioisotopes which is best avoided in pregnancy.

Other tests that may help with the diagnosis include the leukocyte alkaline phosphatase score, bone marrow aspirate, biopsy, cytogenetics and erythropoietin assay.

Close liaison with haematologists will be required in cases such as these. Early referral should be made to an obstetric haematology clinic. During pregnancy venesection (i.e. withdrawal of 250–500 ml venous blood) is the most appropriate treatment—the aim is to maintain the haematocrit at less than 45% in primary polycythaemia.

Leucopaenia—low white cells

Low neutrophils are the greatest concern. A neutrophil count less than $1.0 \times 10^9/l$ puts the patient at significantly increased risk of infection. These patients should be referred urgently to a combined haematology/obstetric clinic. Repeat the FBC in the first instance to confirm. Blood film examination/comment is important. Ethnic origin influences the neutrophil count. Afro-Caribbean races tend to have a lower peripheral neutrophil count—this is not associated with any disease and is due to an increase in neutrophil margination. Low neutrophils can occur acutely or chronically, as an isolated finding or part of a generalised pancytopaenia (i.e. a DECREASE in all of the cellular components of the blood). Neutropenia may be due to peripheral destruction or an underlying bone marrow disease. Any implicated drugs should be stopped if the neutropenia is severe. The blood film and patient should be examined and a bone marrow investigation considered if no cause is obvious.

Leucocytosis—high white cell count

A high white cell count is most likely to be reactive, i.e. secondary to infection or inflammation. It can also be associated with pre-eclampsia, haemorrhage and malignant disease. A persistently raised white cell count that does not settle in the postpartum period should be further investigated to rule out chronic myeloid leukaemia. A leucocyte alkaline phosphatase score can be arranged with the haematology laboratory and can be helpful in distinguishing this, as in reactive conditions it is elevated but in chronic myeloid leukaemia it is low.

Thrombocytopenia—low platelet count

A low platelet count should be confirmed in the first instance with a repeat sample. The blood film should be examined to ensure there is no platelet clumping. Having ascertained the low count is real, the timing of its occurrence and whether it was present outside of pregnancy provide diagnostic clues. The most common reason for thrombocytopenia in pregnancy is gestational or incidental thrombocytopenia. This usually occurs in the third trimester and only occasionally in the second trimester. Platelet counts generally do not fall below $70 \times 10^9/l$. The cord and neonatal platelet counts are normal and the mother's platelet count recovers in the postpartum period. Hypertensive disorders of pregnancy can be associated with thrombocytopenia (accounts for 20–25% thrombocytopenic pregnant women). Immune thrombocytopenia is a diagnosis of exclusion. It can present in any trimester with any level of platelet count. A low cord or neonatal platelet count and failure of the maternal count to recover in the postpartum period support the diagnosis.

Platelet counts of less than $100 \times 10^9/l$ should be referred to a specialist obstetric haematology clinic for further assessment.

Thrombocytosis—high platelet count

A high platelet count is most likely to be reactive, i.e. secondary to infection or inflammation. It can also be associated with pre-eclampsia, haemorrhage and malignant disease. A persistently raised platelet count that does not settle requires further investigation. A platelet count of more than $600 \times 10^9/l$ that persists for more than 6 weeks without obvious explanation requires further specialist haematological investigation and these women should be referred to a specialist obstetric haematology clinic.

Points for discussion with parents

- Reason for screening full blood counts—information about haemoglobin, white cells and platelets
- The timing of FBCs and when and how the results will be given to the woman
- Prevention of iron deficiency anaemia:
  - Dietary advice
  - Prophylactic iron supplements if at risk
- Periconceptual folic acid
- That all tests will only be performed with the consent of the woman.

Points for discussion with parents if relevant

■ Explanation of any abnormality in the FBC, follow-up investigations required, and, if necessary, referral to an obstetric haematology clinic

■ How iron deficiency is treated

■ Side effects of iron tablets.

Clinical scenario (Box 4.1)

Box 4.1 Clinical scenario

A 30-year-old Indian lady is admitted under the medical team. She is 8 weeks pregnant. She has 5 children under the age of 6, is vegetarian and enjoys chapattis and tea.

Results

Haemoglobin	6 g/dl
White cell count	6×10^9/l
Platelets	170×10^9/l
MCV	53
MCH	14

Blood film comment: poikilocytosis, pencil cells
Hypochromic, microcytic red cells

Ferritin	1 µg/l

Haemoglobin electrophoresis normal

Results 3 weeks after treatment

Haemoglobin	9 g/dl
White cell count	6×10^9/l
Platelets	170×10^9/l
MCV	65
MCH	19

Blood film comment dimorphic

QUESTIONS

1. What type of anaemia does this lady have?
2. What are her risk factors for this type of anaemia?
3. Is the haemoglobin electrophoresis result absolute reassurance there is no haemoglobinopathy?
4. What haemoglobinopathies could this lady have?
5. What strategies could one adopt to deal with this?
6. What treatment has this lady had?
7. What are the treatment options?

ANSWERS

1. Iron deficiency anaemia
2. Multiparity, several pregnancies over a short period, diet—vegetarianism and the tea and phytates in chapattis inhibit iron absorption.
3. No, it is not absolute reassurance.
4. She could have an alpha (α) thalassaemia trait or beta (β) thalassaemia trait with a normal HbA_2 because of the iron deficiency.
5. Strategies to deal with this include treating the iron deficiency and then repeating the screen and carrying out a haemoglobinopathy screen on the husband.
6. This lady has had oral iron therapy—the dimorphic blood film indicates two populations of red cells: poorly haemoglobinised iron deficient cells and normal iron replete red cells.
7. Treatment options include oral or parenteral iron. Blood transfusion should be avoided as this is a chronic anaemia and the woman has compensated for this.

HAEMOGLOBINOPATHY SCREENS[5]

Haemoglobinopathies are inherited disorders of haemoglobin. Haemoglobin is made up of four globin chains and haem (a combination of iron and porphyrin). There are different types of globin chain at different stages of development and in adulthood there are three different types of haemoglobin present (Table 4.4). When there are abnormalities in the quantity or quality of globin chains the resulting conditions are known as haemoglobinopathies.

The *quantitative* abnormalities (i.e. *number* of globin chains produced is reduced) are known as the thalassaemia syndromes. Alpha (α) thalassaemia results from reduced alpha (α) chain production (Table 4.5) and beta (β) thalassaemia results from reduced beta (β) chain production (Table 4.6).

The sickling disorders are *qualitative* abnormalities, i.e. the *quality* (or function) of the globin

Table 4.4 Normal adult haemoglobins

Haemoglobin	Globin chain makeup	Adult	Pregnant female
HbA	2 alpha chains (α) 2 beta chains (β) = $\alpha_2\beta_2$	95–98%	Unchanged
HbA2	2 alpha chains (α) 2 delta chains (δ) = $\alpha_2\delta_2$	1.8–3.4%	Unchanged
HbF	2 alpha chains (α) 2 gamma chains (γ) = $\alpha_2\gamma_2$	Approximately 1%	A physiological rise is seen in 15–24% of pregnant women. HbF can rise up to 5% and this occurs in the second trimester

Table 4.5 Alpha thalassaemia

Phenotype	Number of functional alpha genes	Genotype	Red cell indices abnormalities	Significance	Electrophoresis abnormalities
Normal	4	$\alpha\alpha/\alpha\alpha$	Normal	Normal	Normal
Mild alpha thalassaemia trait	3	$-\alpha/\alpha\alpha$	Normal	No clinical significance. If partner has 2 alpha gene deletion, fetus at risk of HbH	Normal
Severe alpha thalassaemia trait	2	$-\alpha/-\alpha$ $--/\alpha\alpha$	Hypochromic, microcytic Suspect if MCH less than 25 pg	If double gene deletion inherited from 1 parent and partner, the same 1:4 risk of hydrops fetalis (see text)	Normal
HbH disease	1	$--/-\alpha$	Hypochromic, microcytic	Chronic haemolytic anaemia with normal life expectancy	Raised HbH 2–40% usually 8–10%). Hb Bart's is sometimes present (up to 5%) Reduced HbA_2 and raised HbF
Hb Bart's hydrops fetalis (alpha thalassaemia major)	0	$--/--$		Incompatible with life— results in intrauterine hydrops	Haemoglobin Bart's and sometimes smaller amounts of embryonic haemoglobins and HbH

Table 4.6 Beta thalassaemia

Phenotype	Number of functional beta genes	Example of possible genotype	Red cell indices abnormalities	Significance	Electrophoresis abnormalities
Normal	2	β/β	Normal	Normal	Normal
Beta thalassaemia trait	Usually 1 but less than 2	β/β^0 β/β^+	Hypochromic, microcytic anaemia (mild)	If both parents have only 1 beta gene then 1:4 chance of β thalassaemia major	Elevated HbA2 Greater than 3.5%
Beta thalassaemia intermedia	Usually less than 1 but more than nil	β^+/β^0 Diverse genetic subtleties	Moderate hypochromic, microcytic anaemia	If mother and partner carry a β^0 gene then 1:4 chance of β thalassaemia major	Elevated HbA2 more than trait and raised HbF
Beta thalassaemia major	Nil	β^0/β^0	Severe anaemia	If partner has β^0 thalassaemia trait then 1:2 chance of β thalassaemia major	HbA absent HbF 98% HbA2 2%

Key:
β normal beta gene—normal globin chain synthesis
β^+ decreased, partial beta gene—reduced but not absent globin chain synthesis
β^0 absent beta gene—absent globin chain synthesis

chains is reduced. Abnormal or variant haemoglobin is produced because of an amino acid substitution in the α or β globin chain. There are many different types of haemoglobin that sickle—over 300 abnormal variants are recognised.

Antenatal haemoglobinopathy screening[6,7]

Screening for haemoglobinopathies antenatally is in the process of becoming universal in many parts of the UK. This means it is independent of any visual or verbal judgements about ethnicity. Currently screening is undertaken on the basis of family origin, or universally in areas of high incidence.

It is recognised that screening for haemoglobinopathies must be undertaken early enough to allow parents a full choice of options. In reality, for many women this means that a full assessment of

risk with further testing if needed must be completed before the end of the first trimester. Uptake rates for fetal testing are strongly linked to the gestation at which the potential problem is identified with many parents feeling unable to consider a termination after 12 weeks.

Women with full blown haemoglobinopathies should already be known to haematologists and should be referred for early booking. These include women with sickling disorders or thalassaemia intermedia or major. These women are likely to be under active haematological follow-up and it is important that they are closely managed by experienced obstetricians with an interest in conjunction with haematologists. Screening of partners for haemoglobinopathy traits is important because if the partner has a relevant heterozygous condition, the risk of an affected fetus is 1:2.

Screening is designed to detect people who are haemoglobinopathy carriers. Centres usually have a specific antenatal haemoglobinopathy screening request form. Every effort should be made to use these and to fill in appropriate details such as gestation, ethnic origin and partner details.

What makes up a haemoglobinopathy screen?

1. A blood sample in EDTA for haemoglobin electrophoresis, isoelectric focusing or high performance liquid chromatography: Different haemoglobins can be separated out and quantified using these methods. Abnormal or variant haemoglobins can also be detected and quantified.
2. Iron estimation: This is important as iron deficiency can affect the haemoglobinopathy results and make interpretation of red cell indices difficult.
3. FBC: The haemoglobin, red cell count, red cell indices and blood film can add important diagnostic information.
4. Confirmatory test if variant haemoglobin detected: This is initiated by the laboratory, e.g. sickle solubility test for sickling haemoglobins.

Thalassaemia traits may be suspected in women who have hypochromic microcytic indices (i.e. reduced MCH and MCV) on a full blood count that have no other explanation (i.e. there is no iron deficiency).

Alpha thalassaemia

In people with α thalassaemia trait there are no other abnormalities on routine haemoglobinopathy screening. Confirmation can only be made by DNA testing in a regional centre.

α thalassaemia major is a disorder of intrauterine life. It is incompatible with life and results in intrauterine hydrops. Antenatal screening for α thalassaemia is aimed at preventing haemoglobin Bart's hydrops. This can occur when women and their partners have two alpha gene deletions (i.e. genotype —/αα or α^0 thalassaemia trait). In these partnerships there is a 1:4 chance of a hydropic fetus. As α thalassaemia alone does not cause any haemoglobin electrophorectic abnormality, the finding of unexplained hypochromic microcytosis warrants further investigation.

- A mean corpuscular haemoglobin (MCH) concentration of less than 25 pg in an 'at risk' racial group should prompt partner testing.

- DNA analysis should be performed if the partnership appears at risk.
- The 'at risk' racial groups for α^0 thalassaemia trait are the Chinese, South East Asians and Mediterraneans.

Beta thalassaemia

In the majority of patients with β thalassaemia trait there is a raised HbA2 in addition to the hypochromic indices. Haemoglobin variants will be detected by electrophoresis, isolelectric focusing or high performance liquid chromatography and there will be a comment on the report.

β thalassaemia major is a disease of extrauterine life. Infants are well at birth as they are protected by residual fetal haemoglobin. As this fetal haemoglobin wanes, anaemia develops and this becomes progressively more severe. A child that is inadequately transfused at this stage will have stunted growth and develop marrow expansion leading to bossing of the skull, expanded maxilla and other skeletal abnormalities. Eventually other organs can become affected, particularly as a result of iron deposition, and death will ensue usually by 10 years of age. Children who receive transfusions will grow and develop normally. These are required every 4–6 weeks for life and carry risks such as transfusion reactions, red cell alloimmunisation, infections and iron overload. To avoid iron overload, children on transfusion regimens require iron chelation with subcutaneous desferrioxamine in a pump over 12 hours each night for 5–7 days a week. This is normally required from about the age of 2 onwards.

Antenatal screening in β thalassaemia is aimed at preventing or at least detecting β thalassaemia major. In order to do this it is important to detect β thalassaemia trait or heterozygote state.

- Racial groups at most risk include those of Mediterranean origin and also some Asian populations. It can, however, occur in any racial group. Cyprus has a high carrier rate at 1:7 compared with a rate of 1:10 000 in the UK.
- β thalassaemia trait does not cause any clinical symptoms.
- It does not affect the mother's health.
- It is usually suspected due to hypochromic microcytic red cell indices on an FBC and diagnosed by a raised HbA2 on haemoglobin electrophoresis.

It is important to remember that β thalassaemia trait can cause hypochromic, microcytic indices and therefore to ensure that any prescribed iron therapy is based on measurements *of iron stores* rather than FBC alone. It is also important to note that severe iron deficiency can bring the HbA2 into the normal range in a person with β thalassaemia trait, such that the diagnosis can be missed if women are severely iron deficient. Any woman with an MCH less than 27 pg on their FBC should have HbA2 checked. If this is greater than 3.5 this indicates the woman has β thalassaemia trait and her partner should be screened to determine the risk of a child being affected with a major haemoglobinopathy. If the HbA2 is normal in an iron deficient mother from a high-risk group, iron supplementation may be given and the electrophoresis repeated once the mother is iron replete. In practice this can lead to considerable delay in establishing the true picture, and partner testing should be considered where there is a high index of suspicion of β thalassaemia trait in the mother.

If the mother carries a β thalassaemia trait and the partner carries any of the following:

- sickle cell trait
- β thalassaemia trait
- haemoglobin E

there is a 1:4 risk of a major haemoglobinopathy. Sickle cell/β thalassaemia is a major sickling disorder whereas haemoglobin E/β thalassaemia and homozygous β thalassaemia are transfusion dependent states with all the associated problems of iron overload and iron chelation therapy.

Other haemoglobin variants

As previously stated, an abnormal or variant haemoglobin is produced because of an amino acid substitution in an α or β globin chain. There are many different variant haemoglobins—not all are clinically significant. The haemoglobins are named after letters in the alphabet or the places where they were discovered. There are many different haemoglobins that sickle and it important to recognise carriers of significant variant haemoglobins that when inherited with sickle haemoglobin will cause a sickle cell disease. Antenatal screening is aimed at detecting partnerships that are at risk of having a child with a major sickling disease.

Sickle cell haemoglobinopathies

Sickling diseases are multisystem disorders. Sickle cell disease and traits are more common in people of African-Caribbean and sub-Saharan African origin. The common variants causing sickle cell problems are HbS and HbC.

Patients who are homozygous for HbS (i.e. HbSS), or who carry one HbS and one HbC gene, are said to have sickle cell disease. These diseases are marked by periods of wellbeing interspersed with episodes of deterioration. Sickling of red cells occurs with deoxygenation. Sickling causes haemolysis. The sickled cells lodge in the microcirculation causing vaso-occlusion, hypoxia and ischaemia. The ischaemia leads to pain with tissue death. This is known as a painful or vaso-occlusive crisis. There are other types of crisis including aplastic, sequestration and haemolytic.

- Aplastic crisis occurs when red cell production is suppressed. Infection with parvovirus B19 and also folic acid deficiency can cause this. Clinically there is a dramatic fall in haemoglobin. Usually there is a high turnover of red cells in this haemolytic state. Even a temporary reduction in red cell production results in a rapid fall in haemoglobin.
- Sequestration crises occur in children or occasionally adults with an enlarged spleen. There is sudden massive pooling of red blood cells in the spleen resulting in hypotension and even death.
- Haemolytic crises occur due to a rapidly increased rate of haemolysis.

Aside from crises patients have a chronic haemolytic anaemia and increased susceptibility to infection and organ damage where sickling occurs. The severity of symptoms varies widely. Women with sickle cell trait are generally well and usually have a haemoglobin within or at the lower end of the normal range.

Partner screening should be undertaken in all women who carry sickle cell trait or who have sickle cell disease, as there are a large number of haemoglobin variants that can cause problems to a child in combination with HbS.

Discussion points with parents[7]

Discussion centres around the issues of informed consent. Parents need pre test information. Mothers should receive an information booklet in their language as early as possible. Parents need to understand the purpose of the haemoglobinopathy screen, what is being tested for and what the test involves. This will involve discussion about the nature and effects of haemoglobinopathies, how and when test results will be available, the meaning of the results and how a fetal diagnosis would be obtained. Options following a positive fetal diagnosis, the consequences for life and how further information can be obtained also need to be covered.

Mothers should be allowed time to consider screening if they wish and they should be provided with contacts for further discussion. Interpreters should be made available if the mother does not understand English.

All discussions and screening decisions should be documented in the hand-held records.

Guidance interpreting results and subsequent actions (Fig. 4.2)

The basic rule interpreting results is that if the woman has a full blown haemoglobinopathy or any trait, the partner needs urgent haemoglobinopathy testing and testing should not be decided on ethnic origin. Screening of the partner should be undertaken without delay. Subsequent actions depend on the partner's results. If the couple are at risk of having a baby with a major haemoglobinopathy, urgent referral should be made to a combined obstetric and haematology clinic. Counselling will include:

- the potential outcomes of the pregnancy
- the risk of an affected fetus
- the possibility of antenatal diagnosis, including discussion about the risks and timing of this
- potential options should the fetus be found to have inherited a major or life-threatening disorder.

If the partner is unavailable then discussion may entail potential risks based on the racial origin of the partner and background carrier rates for the major variants.

As previously mentioned, the uptake of further testing in an at-risk partnership is integrally related to the gestation at which the potential risk is defined. From 70 to 95% of women will request

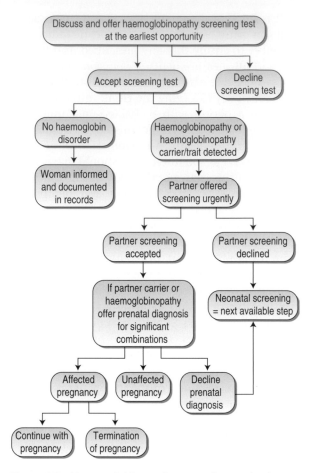

Figure 4.2 Haemoglobinopathy screening and subsequent actions.

further testing if this can be done in the first trimester. In some cultures, termination of pregnancy is only an option before 12 weeks' gestation.

At each stage the woman should be informed and the relevant information documented in the notes.

Antenatal haemoglobinopathy action points

1. Any woman with the following major haemoglobinopathies should be referred to the obstetric haematology clinic for care during pregnancy:
   a. Sickle cell anaemia (HbSS)
   b. Hb SC disease

c. Hb S/β thalassaemia
d. Hb S/D Punjab
e. Hb S/O Arab
f. Hb S/HPFH
g. β thalassaemia major
h. β thalassaemia intermedia
i. Hb H disease
j. Hb E/β thalassaemia
k. Hb SE
l. Hb S/Lepore.

2. Maternal conditions requiring partner testing:
   a. The major haemoglobinopathies listed above in 1
   b. Carrier states (traits) in mother:
      (i) Hb AS
      (ii) Hb AC
      (iii) Hb AD Punjab
      (iv) Hb AE
      (v) Hb AO Arab
      (vi) Hb ALepore
      (vii) δβ thalassaemia trait
      (viii) β thalassaemia trait
      (ix) α^0 thalassaemia trait
      (x) HPFH
      (xi) Any compound heterozygote states including one or more of the above.

3. Couples who require urgent referral to the next antenatal clinic for discussion about prenatal diagnosis if any of the following are present in both:
   a. The major haemoglobinopathies listed above in 1
   b. Carrier states (traits):
      (i) α^0 thalassaemia trait
      (ii) β thalassaemia trait
      (iii) δβ thalassaemia trait
      (iv) Hb AS
      (v) Hb AC
      (vi) Hb AD
      (vii) Hb AE
      (viii) Hb AO Arab
      (ix) Hb ALepore
      (x) HPFH
      (xi) Unstable haemoglobins.

4. Significant fetal haemoglobinopathies—the occurrence of which should be predicted:
   a. Haemoglobin Bart's hydrops fetalis (α^0/α^0)
   b. β thalassaemia major and intermedia including HbE/β thalassaemia

5. Sickle cell disease:
   a. Sickle cell anaemia (Hb SS)
   b. Sickle cell/haemoglobin C disease (Hb SC)
   c. Sickle cell/β thalassaemia (β^0, β^+, δβ thalassaemia)
   d. Sickle cell/haemoglobin Lepore (HbS/Lepore)
   e. Sickle cell/haemoglobin D Punjab (HbSD Punjab)
   f. Sickle cell/haemoglobin O Arab (HbO Arab)

Clinical scenario

Box 4.2 Clinical scenario

An Asian lady in a consanguineous marriage is 8 weeks pregnant in her second pregnancy.

Her blood results

FBC:		
Hb	11.2	
White cell count	5.2	
Platelets	224	
Mean corpuscular volume (MCV)	63	
Mean corpuscular haemoglobin (MCH)	20	
Ferritin		20 ug/l
Haemoglobin electrophoresis	HbA2	6.1%
	HbF	1.6%

Her husband's results

FBC:		
Hb	13.2	
White cell count	6.6	
Platelets	276	
Mean corpuscular volume (MCV)	59	
Mean corpuscular haemoglobin (MCH)	18	
Haemoglobin electrophoresis	HbA2	5.3%
	HbF	0.7%

QUESTIONS

1. Does this lady require iron therapy?
2. What is her diagnosis?
3. Look at the husband's blood results—what is your interpretation of these?
4. What are the implications for this pregnancy?

ANSWERS

1. She does not require iron therapy—her haemoglobin and ferritin are adequate. The hypochromic microcytic indices are secondary to a haemoglobinopathy trait.
2. The raised HbA2 indicates this lady has β thalassaemia trait.
3. The husband has microcytic hypochromic red cell indices with a raised HbA2, indicating he too carries β thalassaemia trait.
4. This couple have a 1:4 chance of having a child affected with β thalassaemia and should be referred urgently to the next combined obstetric haematology clinic for counselling and the offer of antenatal diagnosis.

THROMBOPHILIA SCREENS[8]

Thrombophilia screens are a set of blood tests analysed by coagulation +/− genetic laboratories and immunology to test for underlying hypercoagulable states. These screens are comprised of 6–8 different tests. The majority of the tests are assessing inherited prothrombotic factors. These include levels of the natural anticoagulants protein C and protein S and antithrombin activity. Other inherited tests include activated protein C resistance, factor V Leiden mutation (fVL) and the prothrombin gene mutation (PT20210). Antiphospholipid antibodies are acquired disorders associated with thrombosis. Tests for antiphospholipid antibodies include lupus anticoagulant (tested in the coagulation laboratory on a citrate sample) and anticardiolipin antibodies (tested in the immunology laboratory on a clotted sample).

Deficiency of protein C, S or antithrombin, the presence of factor V Leiden, the prothrombin gene mutation and antiphospholipid antibodies all predispose to venous thrombosis (and arterial thromboses in the case of antiphospholipid antibodies).

Venous thromboembolism is an important cause of maternal mortality and morbidity. Pregnancy and the puerperium are times of increased risk for venous thromboembolism—this is physiological and due to the following factors:

- Relaxation of the vascular smooth muscle
- Compression of the pelvic veins leading to decreased venous return to the vena cava

- Changes in the clotting system and feedback mechanisms:
  - procoagulant proteins increase
  - some of the body's natural anticoagulants decrease
  - impaired fibrinolysis (clot digestion)
- In addition there may be other acquired risk factors such as immobility, dehydration, obesity, Caesarean section, age (over 35 years) and intercurrent medical conditions (e.g. pre-eclampsia or renal disease).

Universal screening of all pregnant women for thrombophilia is not justified. This approach is unlikely to be cost effective and the natural history of thrombophilia in pregnancy is not established, especially in women who are asymptomatic. Additionally, the need for and type of interventions in this situation are unknown.

Women are asked at booking if they have a personal and/or family history of venous thromboembolism (deep vein thrombosis or pulmonary embolus). Women with a positive personal or family history usually have thrombophilia screens carried out. Around half of these women will have a definable thrombophilic defect (see Table 4.7). Some asymptomatic women will enter into pregnancy knowing they have a thrombophilia, having already been tested as part of family screening.

Thrombophilia screening results may aid antenatal, peripartum and postpartum anticoagulation management decisions and can assist thrombotic risk stratification of women. The clinical history, however, is of paramount importance and lack of definable thrombophilia does not mean lack of thrombotic risk. For example, a woman who has a spontaneous pulmonary embolus in her twenties and a negative thrombophilia screen would be considered to be at medium to high risk of a venous thromboembolic event in pregnancy and worthy of antenatal and postpartum heparin prophylaxis. Compare this with a 24-year-old woman who has been screened for thrombophilia and found to be a factor V Leiden heterozygote because a 60-year-old aunt had a deep vein thrombosis after a hip operation. Despite the positive thrombophilia screen, she has no personal history of thrombosis and her family history of thrombosis is in association with an operation. There is no family history of

Table 4.7 Interpreting thrombophilia screens and subsequent actions

Parameter	Normal non-pregnant range (guide—will vary between laboratories)	Changes in pregnancy	Classification of abnormal results	Diagnostic significance of this thrombophilia
Antithrombin	>80 iu/dl	Stable levels, not significantly affected	Low levels—antithrombin deficiency	High-risk thrombophilia
Protein C	>75 iu/dl	No change	Low levels—protein C deficiency	Moderate-risk thrombophilia
Protein S	55–120 iu/dl	Falls progressively in pregnancy—range for pregnancy not well established	Low levels—protein S deficiency or physiological decrease in protein S Interpret results with caution Seek haematological advice	Low/moderate-risk thrombophilia
Activated protein C resistance (APCR)—clotting marker for factor V Leiden	>1.8	Can reduce independent of factor V Leiden	Low levels—activated protein C resistance	Usually indicative of factor V Leiden. Heterozygotes—low-risk thrombophilia
Factor V Leiden mutation	Range does not apply—mutation either present or absent If present patient either heterozygote or homozygote	No change	Factor V Leiden heterozygote or factor V Leiden homozygote	Heterozygotes—low-risk thrombophilia. Homozygotes—moderate-risk thrombophilia
Prothrombin gene mutation PT 20210	Range does not apply—mutation either present or absent If present patient either heterozygote or homozygote	No change	Either heterozygote or homozygote for the mutation	Heterozygotes—low-risk thrombophilia Homozygotes—moderate-risk thrombophilia
Antiphospholipid antibodies: lupus anticoagulant Anticardiolipin antibodies	Range does not apply—the antibodies are either present or absent	No change	Either lupus anticoagulant positive and/or anticardiolipin antibodies present in low, moderate or high titre	High-risk thrombophilia

pregnancy-associated venous thromboembolic events. This woman would be considered to be at low risk of a venous thromboembolic event. Heparin prophylaxis would be given if she had additional acquired risk factors such as a Caesarean section. Heparin prophylaxis would be considered for 6 weeks in the postpartum period.

The importance of individual assessment of these women with regard to their personal and family history of venous thrombosis can not be over emphasised. It is very important to assess the severity and circumstances (spontaneous or acquired) of previous thrombotic events and acquired risk factors, and whether these are still present. The effect of inherited factors or antiphospholipid antibodies must be considered in the light of the woman's past medical history. This is best done in a combined obstetric haematology clinic where decisions can be made about anticoagulant protocols for pregnancy, the peripartum period and the puerperium. Women are counselled about the use of subcutaneous low-molecular-weight heparin, the potential side effects, and they are taught to give the injections in this setting. They are then monitored throughout the pregnancy. It is important to refer women with thrombophilia and/or a significant personal or family history for an individual assessment.

In addition to the potential maternal risk there is some (though not conclusive) evidence that thrombophilias may increase the risk of conditions such as intrauterine growth restriction, pre-eclampsia and fetal loss. The family and obstetric history will be helpful in evaluting the risk in the index pregnancy.

Discussion points with parents

Mothers need to understand the purpose of the thrombophilia screen and its limitations. This will involve discussion about venous thromboembolism, the increased risk of this in pregnancy and the puerperium, and how risk assessments are made on an individual basis depending on the woman's personal and family history of venous thrombosis. She needs to understand what the test involves and how and when test results will be available, and also the meaning of the results. Management decisions should be made after dis-

cussion with the woman concerned and other members of her family, if appropriate. As far as possible her views should be incorporated in management plans.

Interpreters should be made available if the mother does not understand English.

COAGULATION SCREENS[9]

Coagulation screens are performed for many reasons. They can be done to diagnose coagulation disorders, to screen for disorders and also to monitor anticoagulant therapy. Midwives often become involved in taking coagulation screens and passing on results in the emergency situation of disseminated intravascular coagulation. Testing outside of this setting will usually occur in specialist combined obstetric haematology clinics.

To understand coagulation screens it is useful to have a little understanding of the coagulation cascade.

The process of blood coagulation is a series of steps which finally result in the formation of a fibrin clot. Blood coagulation is a result of the activation of either the relatively slow intrinsic pathway or the faster extrinsic pathway. Both these pathways have different clotting factors (denoted by Roman numerals) within them that are activated in a cascade fashion. Both pathways activate factor X to factor Xa and the pathway is then the same from this point to clot formation. This is known as the common pathway. Different coagulation tests reflect specific parts of the coagulation pathway.

The normal ranges quoted for these tests are normal adult ranges and not those for a pregnant female population. Physiological changes in pregnancy cause many of the coagulation factors to increase (e.g. II, VII, VIII, X and fibrinogen) and this is reflected in results of the screening tests.

Disseminated intravascular coagulation (DIC)[10,11]

In this clinical syndrome bleeding manifestations usually predominate. There is widespread activation of the clotting system. This leads to fibrin (clot) formation in small- and medium-sized blood vessels and the consumption and depletion of clotting factors. The body also consumes platelets and activates the fibrinolytic system.

DIC is a symptom and not a disease in itself. Treatment of DIC is aimed at the underlying disorder responsible for it, correcting the coagulopathy and restoring and maintaining blood volume. Obstetric complications that are associated with DIC include:

- Placental abruption
- Pre-eclampsia and eclampsia
- Amniotic fluid embolism
- Massive obstetric haemorrhage
- Retained dead fetus.

Treatment of the underlying condition in obstetrics usually means immediate termination of the pregnancy.

Laboratory diagnosis of DIC can be made from the simple clotting tests. A full blood count to assess the platelet count and a blood film to look for schistocytes (broken red cells) is also part of a DIC screen. Due to factor consumption, the activated partial thromboplastin time (APTT) and prothrombin time (PT) become abnormally long. Initially, this may be in the normal adult range which at term is prolonged for pregnancy. Fibrinogen values fall but again values in the normal adult ranges should be interpreted with caution since fibrinogen levels are typically increased in pregnancy. Platelets fall and D-dimers rise. D-dimers are a measure of the breakdown of blood clot.

The laboratory tests can guide replacement of blood components. Aggressive correction of the coagulopathy is essential in DIC. This is achieved with the administration of fresh frozen plasma, cryoprecipitate and platelet concentrates. Decisions regarding which blood component should be transfused are based on the values of the APTT, PT and the concentration of fibrinogen and platelets. Fresh frozen plasma replaces factors that have been consumed—this is evident from prolongation of the APTT and PT. Low fibrinogen levels will be replaced by cryoprecipitate and platelets by platelet transfusions. There should be close liaison with the blood bank and a haematologist about replacement blood products. Coagulation screens, including fibrinogen, D-dimers and an FBC, should be repeated regularly to assess ongoing need for blood products and the response to them.

Intravenous fluids and packed red cells are administered as required to maintain the blood volume. In addition to coagulation screens and FBC, a sample and request for cross matching blood is essential

Discussion points with parents

Relatives and the mother, when she has recovered, require debriefing after an episode of DIC. The discussion should explain the reasons it occurred and the treatment necessary, and implications for further pregnancies and how this would be managed.

RED CELL ANTIBODIES AND PREGNANCY[12,13,14]

Antenatal serological testing of maternal blood assesses the ABO and rhesus status and checks for any irregular red cell alloantibodies. Guidelines specify the intervals at which this should take place and this is dependent on the woman's Rhesus type and whether any red cell antibodies are detected. The antenatal blood sampling requesting policy is outlined in Table 4.8.

Red cell antibodies are antibodies against red cell antigens. There are naturally occurring antibodies—the formation of these antibodies does not rely on a sensitising event. Antibodies to the ABO system fall into this category. Alloantibodies against other antigens in the blood group system require stimulation through pregnancy or previous transfusion to be produced. Once an antibody has been identified, it is important that future blood transfusions do not have that antigen. The number and type of antibodies will determine how easy it is to supply compatible blood. Alloantibodies are also of significance in pregnancy as IgG antibodies can cross the placenta and, if the fetal red blood cells carry the antigen the antibody is directed against, they will be destroyed. This can lead to fetal anaemia and in severe cases cause fetal hydrops. Jaundice and kernicterus in the neonatal period are other potential consequences of red cell antibodies.

The clinical purposes of routine serological testing in pregnancy are to identify Rhesus negative women

Table 4.8 Antenatal red cell antibody blood sampling request policy

Rhesus (Rh) type	Antibodies	Sample request
Rh (D) positive	No significant antibodies	Booking and 28 weeks
Rh (D) negative	No significant antibodies	Booking and 28 weeks (should be taken prior to routine anti-D prophylaxis) Delivery
Any Rh (D) type	Anti-D, anti-c, anti-Kell related antibodies	Booking Father of pregnancy 4 weekly until 28 weeks 2 weekly until delivery Delivery (requesting frequency may vary depending upon antibody specificity and/or titre)
Any Rh (D) type	Other significant antibodies	Booking Father of pregnancy 28 weeks Delivery (requesting frequency may vary depending upon antibody specificity and/or titre)

who will be eligible for anti-D immunoglobulin prophylaxis, to ensure provision of compatible blood, and also to identify women with antibodies that put the fetus at risk of haemolytic disease of the newborn (HDNB).

There are many red cell antibodies and it is useful to understand which ones are important causes of HDNB. Red cell antibodies causing HDNB can be broadly classified as follows:

- Antibodies to the Rhesus D antigen. This is the principle cause of severe HDNB.
- Antibodies to other Rhesus antigens other than the D antigen. Anti-c is a common cause of HDNB, especially when combined with anti-E. Other Rhesus antibodies rarely cause HDNB (anti-E alone, anti-C, anti-Cw and anti-e).
- Antibodies to non-Rhesus antigens. Anti-K (Kell) is an important cause of HDNB. This can be severe and is not necessarily related to the strength (titre) of the antibody. In addition to red cell haemolysis it can inhibit fetal red cell production. Other antibodies are known to cause HDNB less commonly and include anti Fya (Duffy), anti Jka (Kidd) and anti-S.
- Antibodies to the ABO system. Group O women have naturally occurring anti-A and anti-B antibodies. These are IgM antibodies that do not cross the placenta. Some group O women pro-

duce immune IgG antibodies when carrying group A or B infants. These IgG antibodies can cross the placenta and cause HDNB. This is usually mild and is not related to the strength (titre) of the antibody.

Although many of the antibodies detected in the antenatal period do not cause HDNB, they may still cause difficulties with cross matching and finding compatible blood.

Management and investigation of potential haemolytic disease

In HDNB due to anti-D, the first aim of management is to prevent antibody development by using prophylactic anti-D routinely, after sensitising events and within 72 hours of delivery if the baby is Rhesus D negative.

An obstetric and transfusion history is useful. The previous obstetric history may give an indication of when intervention is likely to be needed. Haemolytic disease of the newborn tends to be as severe or worse with subsequent pregnancies and as a general rule problems tend to occur approximately 6–8 weeks earlier than in a previously affected pregnancy. Previous intrauterine or neonatal deaths due to HDNB put the pregnancy at very high risk of problems with haemolysis and hydrops.

The transfusion history is also relevant as in some cases the antibody detected may be due to this rather than to pregnancy.

Having detected a significant maternal red cell antibody that can cause HDNB, the next step is to antigen type the partner's red cells with regard to this relevant maternal antibody. It is important that the mother understands that it is the father of the baby that needs to be tested. The antigen typing of the father can help in the prediction of the fetal blood type and therefore the risk of HDNB in this and future pregnancies. If the woman became sensitised during a pregnancy fathered by another partner or by a mismatched blood transfusion, determining the current paternal antigen status is very relevant as the father of the current pregnancy may be negative for the antigen in question. If he is negative for the antigen in question and paternity is assured, further assessment and intervention is unnecessary.

The timings and frequency of the serological testing of antibody titres or dilutions depends on antibody type, partner's blood type, obstetric history and starting titre (see Table 4.9). Test results for anti-D and anti-c are given as the amount of antibody present in the maternal serum in iu/ml. For all other antibodies the results are given as the dilution achieved before there is insufficient antibody to cause red cell clumping. Thus a titre of 1:2 means that after a single dilution there was no clumping. This would be a low level of antibody. A titre of 1:16 states that there were four dilutions before the antibody was too weak to clump cells, implying a much higher level of antibody. It is important to remember that a jump from 1:2 to 1:4 is a single dilution, as is a jump from 1:16 to 1:32

The fetal Rhesus (Rh) status can now be assessed in the sensitised Rh negative mother on a maternal blood sample at 14–16 weeks. It is recognised that fetal DNA is present in the maternal circulation and gene testing can identify whether there is Rh positive DNA present, avoiding the need for invasive testing. This provides an answer with 99.9% certainty when the partner is heterozygous Rh positive (i.e. at 50% risk of producing a Rh positive fetus). Because of heterogenity within the Rh gene the test cannot be 100% certain and so monitoring of Rh D titres must take place even when the fetus has tested Rh negative, but the frequency of testing can be minimised. Testing for other Rh types is not yet available, but this may change in the near future.

Monitoring of the fetus is paramount in pregnancies at risk of HDNB. Where possible this surveillance should be non invasive, using high resolution ultrasound scanning screening for markers of the development of anaemia; increase in middle cerebral artery (MCA) blood velocity and liquor volume; and signs of hydrops including increases in the measurements of liver and heart.

Invasive procedures carry the risk of causing fetal–maternal bleeding which may boost antibody titres.

Determination of fetal antigen status (blood typing) can be carried out by DNA testing on amniocytes.

Amniocentesis is indicated when titres rise above the threshold for fetal blood typing, rise rapidly or there is a suspicious ultrasound, particularly rising maximum velocities on middle cerebral artery (MCA) Doppler analysis. Amniotic fluid can be used not only to type the fetal blood groups, but also to assess the degree of red cell breakdown. Bilirubin in the amniotic fluid produces increased yellowing of the fluid, which can be detected by spectrosopy and compared to standard charts. Serial amniocenteses can provide useful information about fetal anaemia; however, the use of amniocentesis has been almost entirely superseded by the introduction of MCA Doppler analysis.

Fetal blood sampling and intrauterine transfusion is indicated in the assessment and treatment of those fetuses known to be antigen positive who are less than 34 weeks' gestation and are suspected of being significantly anaemic from amniocentesis or ultrasound features. It will also be dictated by the past obstetric history. Delivery is the treatment of choice if significant anaemia occurs at or after 34 weeks' gestation.

At birth a cord blood sample should be sent for haemoglobin estimation, ABO and Rhesus D typing, bilirubin estimation and for a direct antiglobulin test (also known as the direct Coombs test). The direct antiglobulin test (DAT) detects maternal

Table 4.9 Management of red cell antibodies in pregnancy

Red cell antibody	Significant titres	Special features
Anti-D	Less than 4 iu/ml—haemolytic disease of the newborn (HDNB) unlikely 4–15 iu/ml—moderate-risk HDNB More than 15 iu/ml—high-risk HDNB Note: timing of HDNB in previous pregnancies useful guide Rate of titre increase important	Test partner for Rh type. Refer for fetal medicine review Send maternal blood at 14–16 weeks (through fetal medicine centre) if Rh D heterozygous Sequential MCA assessment and fetal transfusion when necessary Anti D prophylaxis available for Rh D negative women: ■ Routinely at 28 & 34 weeks ■ Within 72 hours of birth if child Rhesus positive and no pre-existing anti-D A Kleihauer should be performed to ensure sufficient anti-D given ■ After sensitising events 250 iu before 20 weeks' gestation 500 iu after 20 weeks' gestation A Kleihauer should be performed to ensure sufficient anti-D given
Anti-c	More than 10 iu/ml—moderate-risk HDNB	Nil specific. Similar to anti-D in its behaviour
Anti-K (Kell)	Titres expressed as the dilution at which the antibody still detected. Levels less than 1:16 do not usually cause problems but problems due to anti-K (Kell) antibodies are difficult to relate to the titre—the fetus may be severely affected regardless of titre	Causes fetal/neonatal anaemia by two different methods: ■ Red cell breakdown (haemolysis) ■ Inhibition of red cell production The inhibition of red cell production means optical density measurements on amniotic fluid may be less accurate and anaemic babies are not always DAT positive Approximately 10% of at-risk pregnancies will be severely affected

antibody coating the infant's red cells and can be an indication of HDNB. If the DAT is positive, the baby's serum bilirubin should be measured and the neonatal team should assess the need for phototherapy or exchange transfusion.

Discussion points with parents

Parents need to understand the purpose of blood group and red cell antibody screening, what is being tested for and what the test involves. This will involve discussion about the nature and effects of red cell antibodies, how and when test results will be available, and the meaning of the results. If relevant, the management of significant antibody titres needs to be discussed, including the miscarriage and sensitisation risk of procedures such as amniocentesis and intrauterine transfusion—this would usually be done by the obstetrician managing the pregnancy.

Clinical scenario

A 30-year-old woman, presents as a late booker with no previous antenatal care at 34 weeks' gestation. A previous child had required a blood transfusion at birth but she was unsure of the reason why. She was found to be blood group O Rhesus D positive with a positive antibody screen. The antibody was identified as an anti-c at a level of 12 iu/ml. The ultrasound revealed a small amount of free fluid in the abdomen and a small pericardial effusion. The middle cerebral artery Doppler analysis suggested a significant risk of anaemia. She underwent amniocentesis which showed the amniotic fluid bilirubin estimation was in the high-risk zone.

QUESTIONS

1. What is the diagnosis?
2. What is the management?

ANSWERS

1. The diagnosis is haemolytic disease of the newborn due to an anti-c antibody with signs of fetal hydrops.
2. The amniotic fluid bilirubin level and ultrasound findings indicate that this fetus is in immediate danger. Given the gestational age, early delivery and extra uterine exchange transfusion is the treatment of choice.

CONCLUSION

Testing related to haematological conditions in pregnancy is now quite complex. It is important that mothers understand what is being tested and the implications of this testing. Where there are significant concerns, the advice of the obstetric haematology team should be sought.

References

1. Bain BJ. Normal ranges. In: Bain BJ. Blood cells. 3rd edn. Oxford,UK: Blackwell Science; 1995:147–160.
2. Ramsay M. Maternal values, hematology. In: Ramsay M, James D, Steer P, et al, eds. Normal values in pregnancy. 2nd edn. London: WB Saunders; 2000:33–44.
3. National Institute for Clinical Excellence. Clinical guideline 6. Antenatal care: routine care for the healthy pregnant woman. London: NICE; 2003.
4. James D, Steer P, Weiner CP, et al. High risk pregnancy: management options. 2nd edn. London: WB Saunders; 1999.
5. Bain BJ. Haemoglobinopathy diagnosis. 1st edn. Oxford, UK: Blackwell Science; 2001.
6. Zeuner D, Ades A, Karnon J, et al. Antenatal and neonatal haemoglobinopathy screening in the UK: review and economic analysis. Health Technol Assess 1999; 3(11):1–186.
7. NHS Sickle cell and Thalassaemia Screening Programme 2004 website: www.kclphs.org.uk/haemscreening/antenatal.htm
8. Eldor A. Management of thrombophilia and antiphospholipid syndrome during pregnancy. In: Kitchens CS, Alving BM, Kessler CM, eds. Consultative hemostasis and thrombosis. 1st edn. Philadelphia: WB Saunders; 2002:449–461.
9. Deloughery TG. Tests of hemostasis and thrombosis. In: Deloughery Hemostasis and thrombosis. 1st edn. Texas: Landes Bioscience; 1999:18–27.
10. Bremme K. Haemostasis in normal pregnancy. In: Brenner B, Marder V, Conard J, eds. Women's issues in thrombosis and hemostasis. 1st edn. London: Dunitz; 2002:151–167.
11. Gillis S. Disseminated intravascular coagulation in pregnancy and amniotic fluid embolism. In: Brenner B, Marder V, Conrad J, eds. Women's issues in thrombosis and hemostasis. 1st edn. London: Dunitz; 2002:249–263.
12. British Committee for Standards in Haematology, Blood Transfusion Task Force. Guidelines for blood grouping and red cell antibody testing during pregnancy. Transfusion Medicine 1996; 6:71–74.
13. Royal College of Obstetricians and Gynaecologists, Guidelines and Audit Committee. Use of anti-D immunoglobulin for Rh prophylaxis. Clinical Green Top Guideline (22) 2002. Online. Available: http://www.rcog.org.uk/index.asp?pageID=512.
14. National Institute for Clinical Excellence. Technology appraisal guidance no 41. Guidance on the use of routine antenatal anti-D prophylaxis for RhD-negative women. 2002. Online. Available: http://www.nice.org.uk/page.aspx?o=31679.

5

Maternal diseases in pregnancy

Andrew Simm

INTRODUCTION

In considering maternal diseases in pregnancy, it is important to be aware of the physiological changes that occur in pregnancy, and to have an understanding of diseases outside of pregnancy. Salient features will be highlighted in this chapter, but its purpose is not to act as a medical text. The emphasis is on investigations used in both establishing a diagnosis and, more often, in assessing the impact of the pregnancy on the disease, and the disease on the pregnancy.

Many diseases will be known about before the onset of pregnancy. Referral for consultant-based care is usually appropriate. The referral needs detailed information, and reference to the general practitioner's (GP) records as well as discussion with the GP is appropriate. For example, it is insufficient to refer a patient with Type 1 diabetes without details of the last annual review with the diabetologist or GP. This gives information concerning the quality of diabetes control, type and dose of insulin, and presence or absence of complications that have significance for the pregnancy.

Perhaps the easiest way of looking at this subject is to take the commoner pre-existing diseases that may occur with pregnancy and deal with each in turn.

ENDOCRINE DISEASE: DIABETES

In considering diabetes it is necessary to divide the disease into pre-existing diabetes, whether that is Type 1 or Type 2 diabetes, and gestational diabetes. Type 1 diabetes is an autoimmune condition that destroys the insulin secreting cells of the pancreas, and usually develops in young people. Type 2 diabetes is usually of later and more insidious onset, and is associated with obesity. It represents varying degrees of insulin insensitivity. It may require treatment with insulin, hence the avoidance of the terms insulin and non-insulin dependent diabetes that can be confusing. Gestational diabetes is defined as 'a carbohydrate intolerance of variable severity with onset or first recognition during the present pregnancy'. Thus it may include women with diabetes that was previously unrecognised.

Pre-existing diabetes

Diagnosis outside pregnancy
The diagnosis of frank diabetes relies on finding a diagnostic glucose level as outlined below. These values represent the criteria from the World Health Organisation (WHO):

- If symptomatic, a single raised fasting blood glucose (BG) level ≥ 7.0 mmol/l or ≥ 11.1 mmol/l random.
- If asymptomatic, two fasting venous plasma glucose levels ≥ 7.0 mmol/l or two random venous plasma glucose levels ≥ 11.1 mmol/l.
- Borderline cases should undergo a 75 g oral glucose tolerance test (OGTT) with diagnosis of diabetes made if the fasting BG ≥ 7.0 mmol/l or 2 hour value is ≥ 11.1 mmol/l.

Diabetes is usually known about before the pregnancy, and investigations are aimed at looking for coincidental disease, establishing whether complications are present, and assessing the impact of the disease on the pregnancy and vice versa.

Investigations at booking
In addition to the standard investigations offered to all women at booking, it is advisable to undertake some additional investigations for women with diabetes. These are outlined below:

1. Thyroid function tests (TFTs). Type 1 diabetes and hypothyroidism both have an autoimmune basis, and the prevalence of hypothyroidism in Type 1 diabetes is higher than in the general population.[1] The same is reported to be true for Type 2 diabetes. Normal TFTs at booking do not require repeat testing in the pregnancy.

2. Urea, electrolytes and creatinine. Diabetes can cause nephropathy, and these tests provide a baseline assessment of renal function. If urinalysis reveals persistent proteinuria in the absence of infection, further assessment by a 24-hour urine collection for creatinine clearance and protein quantification is required (see later).

3. HBA1C (glycosylated haemoglobin). This looks at the amount of glucose bound to haemoglobin. It provides an assessment of diabetes control over the preceding month, and ideally should be less than 7%.

4. Since maternal serum screening results are affected by diabetes, many centres offer a nuchal translucency (NT) scan at 11–14 weeks. If NT scanning is not available, the laboratory will adjust for the presence of diabetes on a serum screening test. Hence this information must be included on the test form. It is important to point out that the diabetes does not increase the risk for trisomy 21.

Investigations during pregnancy
Blood glucose monitoring
A blood glucose profile, consisting of preprandial and postprandial (usually 90 minutes) levels, is essential for managing diabetes during pregnancy. Insulin requirements increase significantly as pregnancy progresses, and frequent changes in dose are

required. This can be extremely difficult for the pregnant woman, but is crucial in reducing the complications to the pregnancy, especially miscarriage, congenital malformation, fetal macrosomia and stillbirth.

Glucose levels are ideally between 4 and 6 mmol/l preprandial, and less than 7.5 mmol/l postprandial. Results from blood glucose meters can now be downloaded onto a database in most units. This is important as it is recognised that if sole reliance is given to patient recording, records can be unreliable. This can be for several reasons, often reflecting the woman's willingness to please the physician as well as her family.[2]

Urinalysis

This should be undertaken at each assessment for several reasons:

- Pre-eclampsia is increased in diabetes and thus assessment for proteinuria is important.
- Urinary tract infection is more frequent in pregnancy, and the development of protein or blood in the urine, especially if dysuria is present, should prompt urine culture.
- Microalbuminuria before pregnancy may manifest as overt proteinuria as pregnancy progresses. This reflects nephropathy. Microalbuminuria refers to increased levels of protein in the urine, but not at sufficient levels to cause the dipstick to give a positive reading. Overt proteinuria should prompt protein quantification by way of a 24-hour urine collection. It can be difficult to differentiate from pre-eclampsia, although usually the woman is asymptomatic and not hypertensive. Nephropathy does nonetheless necessitate greater vigilance for the remainder of the pregnancy.
- Ketonuria in the presence of hyperglycaemia is related to poor glucose control in Type 1 diabetes and necessitates urgent hospital review. This may represent developing ketoacidosis that is dangerous for mother and fetus.[3]

Retinal examination

A physician usually undertakes this in each trimester, looking for evidence of diabetic retinopathy. Retinopathy may worsen or appear for the first time in pregnancy, and appears to be related to rapid improvement in glycaemic control. Tropicamide is used to dilate the pupils; hence women are warned not to drive when attending for this assessment. Some women require assessment by an ophthalmic surgeon.

HBA1C

As previously mentioned, this provides some assessment of overall glucose control over the preceding month. It is usually repeated every 4 weeks.

Detailed fetal anomaly scan and fetal echocardiogram (echo)

Congenital malformations, including cardiac, are more common in diabetic pregnancies, and a structural survey including a fetal echo should be undertaken at 20–22 weeks. Undertaking the assessment at this gestation allows the two examinations to be done simultaneously. If the routine anomaly scan does not include a detailed assessment of the fetal heart, this should be arranged separately.

Fetal biometry and liquor assessment

Macrosomia, often accompanied by polyhydramnios, usually reflects poorer diabetes control. Serial biometry allows an assessment of fetal growth over time, and should be used together with glucose control to make an assessment of fetal risk. Macrosomic babies are at increased risk of intrauterine fetal death, presumably because of metabolic disturbance rather than placental dysfunction. Hence umbilical Doppler velocimetry appears less useful for fetal assessment in diabetic pregnancy. Estimation of fetal weight is notoriously inaccurate, especially at this larger end of the scale. Nonetheless, elective lower segment Caesarean section should be considered where the estimated fetal weight exceeds 4500 g in a diabetic pregnancy. This is because the constitution of these babies is different from healthy macrosomic babies, and these babies are particularly at risk of birth trauma. Ultrasound assessment is usually undertaken every 4 weeks from 28 weeks' gestation, but this may need to be more frequent if macrosomia exists. The same is true if growth restriction is evident and this is more common in pregnancies complicated by vascular disease, i.e. with nephropathy or retinopathy. Here umbilical Doppler assessment should be used. In both instances consideration should be given to twice weekly cardiotocograph (CTG) monitoring.

Gestational diabetes mellitus (GDM)

Pregnancy is a diabetogenic state, and glucose tolerance decreases as pregnancy progresses. There is no consensus on who, when or how to screen for diabetes. Fasting glucose levels are normally lower in pregnancy, and postprandial levels higher. However, the cut-offs for diagnosis remain variable. Few would dispute the need for diagnosis and treatment of frank diabetes, as outlined earlier. However, it is likely that with milder levels of glucose intolerance there is a continuum, starting with levels that do not carry a significantly worse prognosis for the pregnancy, continuing through to levels where the fetus is at risk of adverse outcome. Results of multicentre trials are eagerly awaited to try to resolve the issue of what constitutes 'significant glucose intolerance in pregnancy'.

The method of screening varies, but the gold standard is a 75 g glucose tolerance test. Some units use a fasting glucose to determine those who need a full OGTT, with a threshold for continuing to full testing of 6 mmol/l. The WHO criteria are as for the non-pregnant woman but they also give the following definitions:

- Impaired glucose tolerance: fasting plasma glucose <7.0 mmol/l and OGTT 2-hour value ≥7.8 mmol/l but <11.1 mmol/l
- Impaired fasting glycaemia (IFG): fasting plasma glucose ≥6.1 mmol/l but <7.0 mmol/l.

They recommend the use of the term 'gestational diabetes' to encompass frank diabetes and impaired glucose tolerance. Other authorities advise caution with such stringent criteria in pregnancy. It is important to be aware of your own unit's criteria for diagnosis, whilst the results of the large trials are awaited.

Many units use risk factors in deciding whom to screen. These are listed in Box 5.1.

The timing of a glucose tolerance test requires consideration of the risk factors present, but arbitrarily is usually undertaken at 24–28 weeks' gestation. This is based on the premise that glucose intolerance becomes more likely as pregnancy progresses, but allows time for treatment of hyperglycaemia to improve outcome. If there has been previous GDM, it is prudent to screen earlier (12–14 weeks) and repeat the testing later if this is

---

Box 5.1   Risk factors for development of gestational diabetes

- Previous gestational diabetes
- Previous macrosomic baby (again definitions vary, usually birth weight >97th centile for gestation, or more than 4.0–4.5 kg at term)
- First degree relative with diabetes (Type 1 and Type 2)
- Obesity (BMI >35 kg/m^2)
- Suspected large for gestational age fetus in current pregnancy
- Polyhydramnios
- Previous unexplained stillbirth
- Glycosuria*

*The NICE guideline on antenatal care[4] suggests there is no evidence for routine screening for glycosuria. There is widespread debate, for example currently unpublished data from our own unit suggest glycosuria alone was a relatively infrequent risk factor for screening. Nonetheless, it did lead to diagnosis of diabetes in a significant proportion of cases.

---

normal. Multiple risk factors may also lead one to consider doing the same.

Investigations following diagnosis

The diagnosis is usually made in the second or third trimester, and the risk of miscarriage or congenital abnormality attributable to the diabetes is absent. Blood glucose monitoring is usually as for established diabetics, but can be more relaxed in well motivated women who are achieving excellent control by diet alone. HBA1C levels are a useful guide to assess diabetes control. Urinalysis should be as for diabetics, although nephropathy is extremely unlikely in this cohort. Fetal biometry should be undertaken as for established diabetics.

Investigations after delivery

Currently all women with gestational diabetes should have a glucose tolerance test undertaken between 6 and 12 weeks postnatally as some will continue to have impaired glucose tolerance or diabetes. The lifetime risk of developing diabetes in a woman with gestational diabetes is as high as 50%.

ENDOCRINE DISEASE: THYROID

Physiology

The thyroid gland is stimulated by thyroid stimulating hormone from the pituitary gland to produce thyroxine (T4) and triiodothyronine (T3). Most of the body's triiodothyronine (T3) is converted from T4 peripherally. These hormones then feed back to the pituitary to control release and maintain a steady state.

Pregnancy itself affects thyroid function, and reference ranges for thyroid function tests (measurement of free T4, free T3 and thyroid stimulating hormone (TSH)) need establishing for each trimester. Currently non-pregnant reference ranges are frequently used. TSH alone should not be relied upon in pregnancy as this fails to distinguish subclinical hypothyroidism from overt disease. In subclinical hypothyroidism the TSH is raised with a normal T4 (implying the thyroid is 'working harder' to produce sufficient T4) and is usually asymptomatic. In overt hypothyroidism the TSH is raised and T4 reduced.

Hypothyroidism

This is present in approximately 1% of pregnancies, and usually predates the pregnancy. The most common cause in women of reproductive age is autoimmune thyroid disease. Other causes of hypothyroidism include surgery or radioiodine therapy for previous hyperthyroidism. Diagnosis in pregnancy can be difficult as many symptoms are also encountered in normal pregnancy. A family history and the presence of other autoimmune diseases should alert one to consider testing if symptoms are present (see Box 5.2).

Box 5.2   Symptoms of hypothyroidism
■ Fatigue
■ Weight gain
■ Dry skin
■ Coarse dry hair
■ Constipation
■ Cold intolerance
■ Depression

Investigation

Thyroid function tests including TSH and free T4 should be undertaken if there is a clinical suspicion of hypothyroidism, or pregnancy is planned or established in a woman with hypothyroidism. The diagnosis is based on demonstrating a low free T4 in the presence of a raised TSH. Thyroid peroxidase antibodies are useful in confirming an autoimmune aetiology, and should be checked if this has not previously been done. In those already on treatment, the thyroid function tests provide information on the adequacy of replacement therapy.

Importance

Fetal thyroxine production becomes autonomous after the first half of pregnancy, so the fetus relies on maternal thyroxine before this. Small amounts cross the placenta. Given thyroxine is important in neurodevelopment, studies suggest that inadequately treated hypothyroidism results in lower neurodevelopmental scores in the child.[5]

Untreated hypothyroidism also appears to carry a risk to the mother of gestational hypertension and abruption leading to earlier delivery.

Management

Where the diagnosis of hypothyroidism is established, the goal is optimising therapy to keep the TSH below 2.0–2.5 milliunits per litre (miu/l). Ideally this should be achieved pre conception. Further thyroid function tests should be undertaken in the first trimester, and then every 8 weeks, or 4–6 weeks after a change in thyroxine dose. Usually the dose needs increasing in the first half of pregnancy, and then remains stable. If no dose increment is required on testing at 28 weeks, it is usually sufficient to maintain this dose until delivery. The usual advice is then to return to the pre-pregnant dose (assuming good control before conception), and check the TFTs 6 weeks postpartum.

Thyrotoxicosis

This is a clinical syndrome caused by excess circulation of thyroid hormone, and is usually due to thyroid gland overactivity. Other causes include excessive thyroxine ingestion, and hyperemesis gravidarum. In hyperemesis gravidarum, the high levels of human chorionic gonadotrophin (hCG) have thyroid stimulating activity. Usually there is spontaneous resolution as the vomiting settles.

The commonest cause of thyroid overactivity is Grave's disease, with prevalence in pregnancy of 0.1–0.4%. Most cases predate the pregnancy. Again, this is an autoimmune disorder and thyroid peroxidase antibodies are often raised. Specific TSH-receptor stimulating antibodies can be measured but this assay is not widely available and thus not routinely undertaken. These antibodies can cross the placenta and result in fetal or neonatal thyrotoxicosis.

Investigation

Where symptoms suggest thyrotoxicosis, thyroid function tests should be undertaken to confirm or refute this. The diagnosis is confirmed if the T3 or T4 is raised and TSH suppressed (T3 toxicosis may occur before T4 levels rise).

As the stimulating antibodies can cross the placenta, fetal thyrotoxicosis can occur. This is more likely when the mother has been treated by surgery or radiotherapy and is subsequently not requiring anti-thyroid drugs that would also treat the fetus. Fetal tachycardia is the most usual sign and thus fetal heart auscultation should be undertaken at each visit. Ultrasound should be used, if there is suspicion of fetal disease, to look for evidence of growth restriction and a fetal goitre.[6]

Importance

Untreated thyrotoxicosis can result in miscarriage, intrauterine growth restriction, preterm labour, and intrauterine fetal demise. In the mother it can result in a thyroid 'storm' that is potentially life threatening.

Management

If the diagnosis has been established before pregnancy, it is hoped that therapy has been optimised prior to conception. The aim in pregnancy is to achieve T3 and T4 levels towards the top end of the normal range, i.e. using the minimum effective dose of antithyroid drug. These drugs can cross the placenta. Usually the disease goes into remission as the pregnancy progresses, and antithyroid drugs (propylthyouracil or carbimazole) can often be tapered down and stopped. Frequent monitoring (usually every 4 weeks) of TFTs is thus important. If

> **Box 5.3 Signs of neonatal thyrotoxicosis**
>
> - Small for gestational age
> - Thyroid: palpable goitre (diffuse swelling of thyroid gland)
> - Central nervous system: irritability, restlessness
> - Eyes: staring, lid retraction, exophthalmos (abnormal protrusion of eyes)
> - Heart: tachycardia, arrhythmia
> - Gastrointestinal tract: poor weight gain, diarrhoea, vomiting
> - Other: sweatiness, flushing

the pregnant woman stops treatment, there should be vigilance postpartum as recurrence is more common then. Symptoms warrant TFTs; otherwise a check at 6 weeks is sufficient, with regular reassessment over the next 12 months.

1–5% of neonates develop a congenital thyrotoxicosis related to transplacental passage of thyroid stimulating antibodies. It must be remembered that this can occur in babies born to mothers with a history of Grave's disease, such as those previously treated with surgery or radioiodine that may now be hypothyroid and on thyroxine. Women whose babies are at risk should be asked to remain in hospital for 4 days after delivery so the baby can be observed for signs of developing thyrotoxicosis (Box 5.3). The mother should be alerted to the signs of congenital thyrotoxicosis once discharged home.

It is reasonable to breast feed these babies, even if the mother is on propylthiouracil or carbimazole.

Thyroid nodules

Investigation of a thyroid nodule aims to elucidate two facts.

- What is the nature of the lesion?
- Is thyroid function normal?

Thyroid nodules are usually benign, but assessment by an endocrine team is usually warranted. Cystic nodules can be aspirated and fluid sent for cytology. If solid, a needle biopsy can be undertaken.

Thyroid function tests and thyroid peroxidase antibodies should be undertaken to establish whether the woman is euthyroid.

ENDOCRINE DISEASE: PITUITARY

Hyperprolactinaemia

Prolactin levels are increased in normal pregnancy, and thus hyperprolactinaemia referred to here is that predating the pregnancy. Often investigation will already have been undertaken to establish the underlying cause. The commonest of these is a prolactinoma. This refers to a pituitary tumour producing prolactin, and these can be divided by size into macroadenomas (>1 cm) or microadenomas (<1 cm). These are diagnosed by imaging the pituitary gland using magnetic resonance imaging (MRI) or computed tomography (CT). The main concern in pregnancy is tumour growth that is more common with macroprolactinomas.

Prolactin secretion is inhibited by dopamine, thus dopamine agonists (e.g. bromocriptine) are used to treat hyperprolactinaemia. Hyperprolactinaemia causes amenorrhoea, and dopamine agonists are used to restore fertility. Once pregnant, most women can stop treatment. It is sometimes continued in pregnancy in the case of macroadenomas.

Serum prolactin levels are unhelpful in pregnancy. Visual field testing is necessary in women with symptoms of headache or visual field defects, or in those with macroprolactinomas not on therapy. This is because expansion can lead to compression of the optic chiasm. CT or MRI should be undertaken if there is suspicion of tumour expansion.

Breastfeeding is not contraindicated.

Sheehan's syndrome

This is a condition specific to pregnancy where pituitary gland infarction occurs following major postpartum haemorrhage. Complete or partial pituitary failure ensues. The history of a major haemorrhage followed by both failure of lactation and a return to menstruation should lead to investigation including:

- Serum follicle stimulating hormone (FSH) and luteinising hormone (LH)
- Serum oestradiol
- Serum prolactin

- Thyroid function tests (TFTs)
- Serum adrenocorticotropic hormone (ACTH) and cortisol
- Cranial MRI or CT (if abnormalities in any of the above).

HYPERTENSION

Chronic hypertension

This is hypertension predating the pregnancy, but it may only become apparent when a woman's blood pressure is found to be raised in the first half of pregnancy. Chronic hypertension can be classed as:

- Primary (essential) hypertension   90%
- Secondary hypertension   10%
  Causes of secondary hypertension include:
- Renal disease
  - Glomerulonephritis
  - Interstitial nephritis
  - Polycystic kidneys
  - Renal artery stenosis
- Collagen vascular disease (systemic lupus erythematosus)
- Endocrine
  - Diabetes with vasculopathy
  - Phaeochromocytoma
  - Thyrotoxicosis
  - Cushing's disease
  - Hyperaldosteronism (Conn's syndrome)
  - Hyperparathyroidism
- Coarctation of the aorta.[7]

It is important not to assume that hypertension is 'essential' without some basic investigations. Clearly these may have been undertaken before the pregnancy, in which case this information is important to convey to the obstetrician at booking.

Investigations
The initial investigations if hypertension is found in the first half of pregnancy are:

- Urinalysis
  - This determines whether there is underlying proteinuria or haematuria pointing to a renal cause.

- Serum creatinine, urea, electrolytes and calcium:
  - It must be remembered that normal values of creatinine and urea are much lower in pregnancy than in the non-pregnant population
  - Creatinine and urea are important in assessing renal function
  - Hypokalaemia should prompt further investigation into Conn's syndrome
  - High calcium should lead to investigation for hyperparathyroidism.
- Ultrasound scan of the kidneys to exclude:
  - Scarred kidney from chronic pyelonephritis
  - Polycystic kidney disease
  - Renal artery stenosis (Doppler examination of renal artery); this examination is mandatory if there is a renal bruit (flow of blood heard on auscultation over the renal artery).

Further investigation depends on the results of the initial investigations. If proteinuria or haematuria are present, a midstream urine sample should be sent for culture and sensitivity.

If proteinuria persists in the absence of infection, a 24-hour urine collection should be performed. This allows:

- Quantification of the degree of proteinuria
- Assessment of the creatinine clearance, which is a surrogate for the glomerular filtration rate. This assesses renal function, and should also be undertaken if the serum creatinine is raised. Creatinine clearance in pregnancy is usually increased owing to an increased renal blood flow. The method of collection is important (see Box 5.4).

If there is hypokalaemia (serum potassium less than 3 mmol/l), then Conn's syndrome should be considered. Primary hyperaldosteronism can be due to an adrenal adenoma, carcinoma or hyperplasia. The renin/aldosterone ratio is a useful screening test, with an inappropriately raised aldosterone level in the presence of a suppressed renin concentration. The hypokalaemia in the presence of hypertension is not in itself diagnostic of Conn's syndrome.

Phaeochromocytomas are tumours of the adrenal medulla, causing high levels of catecholamines such as adrenaline and noradrenaline. Certainly hypertension in the presence of excessive sweating or palpitations should prompt investigation by

> **Box 5.4   Conducting a 24-hour urine collection**
>
> 1. At the start of the collection the bladder should be emptied and this sample *discarded* (or sent for culture if not already done).
> 2. All urine voided over the next 24 hours should be collected; if any is not the results are invalid.
> 3. After exactly 24 hours the bladder should be emptied and this void should be *included* in the urine collection.
> 4. The start and finish times, together with the date, should be labelled on the bottle so the laboratory technician is aware of the completeness of the collection, and the age of the sample.
> 5. A request card should indicate whether a protein quantification, creatinine clearance, or both, is required.
> 6. 24 hour collections for protein and creatinine clearance can be undertaken using the same sample.
> 7. If a creatinine clearance is being requested a serum creatinine should be sent at the same time as the urine as this is required for the calculation.
> 8. If urinary catecholamines are being requested, a different collection bottle to that used for protein and creatinine clearance must be used as this contains a specific reagent. The woman is advised not to pass urine directly into the bottle as the reagent can be harmful to the skin.

way of a 24-hour urine collection looking for catecholamines. This usually includes measurement of dopamine levels which are affected by the administration of methyldopa. Hence measurement before the commencement of antihypertensives is preferable. If catecholamines are raised, ultrasound or MRI should be undertaken to localise the tumour (10% are extra-adrenal). Although rare, the diagnosis is important as fetal and maternal mortality are significantly increased.

Longstanding hypertension is not frequently encountered in pregnancy, although with later childbearing it is becoming more common. Usually these women will have been fully investigated before pregnancy. In this group investigation should include assessment of end-organ damage:

- Electrocardiogram (ECG)
- Echocardiogram (Echo)
- Retinal assessment
- Creatinine clearance.

Women with chronic hypertension are at increased risk of developing pre-eclampsia.

Drug treatment and chronic hypertension
Many women with chronic hypertension will be on antihypertensive medication. Whilst some therapies are contraindicated in pregnancy, none are teratogenic in the first trimester. There is usually time to find an alternative. The following medicines are usually discontinued:

- Angiotensin converting enzyme (ACE) inhibitors and angiotensin II inhibitors (these preparations often end in 'pril', for example captopril). These cause fetal renal impairment and must be stopped by 12–14 weeks (i.e. when fetal renal function commences).
- Atenolol. This is a beta blocker. At doses of 100 mg per day, significant fetal growth restriction may be seen. Other beta blockers and combined alpha and beta blockers (for example, labetalol) appear to cause fewer problems. The growth restriction is usually after 24 weeks. Some women take atenolol for other reasons (for example, as an antidysrhythmic). They may need to continue, as this is highly effective.
- Diuretics. These can cause electrolyte disturbance and are usually discontinued.

Labetalol and methyldopa are often used as first line treatment in pregnancy. Nifedipine is often added if these do not adequately control hypertension.

Pre-eclampsia

Pre-eclampsia, although diagnosed on the basis of hypertension and proteinuria after the 20th week of pregnancy, is a multisystem disorder that carries risk to both mother and fetus. Its presentation is varied, affecting mother and fetus to varying degrees and at varying stages of pregnancy. It is now considered to represent an excessive systemic inflammatory response, triggered by a placental factor (as yet unknown), and revealed in those

women with a predisposition to the inflammatory burden.[8]

Diagnosis is not always easy. It is distinguished from pregnancy-induced hypertension (PIH) by the absence of proteinuria and other systemic features. Pregnancy-induced hypertension carries a good prognosis, but requires regular surveillance to identify those women who are in the process of developing pre-eclampsia. It is important to ask about symptoms of headache, visual disturbance and epigastric pain. Oedema should be noted although it is so common in pregnancy it has been removed from the definition of pre-eclampsia. The symphyseal fundal height should be measured.

Investigation of the woman with suspected pre-eclampsia should include:

- Full blood count (FBC). Thrombocytopenia (low platelets) can occur.
- Urea, creatinine and electrolytes. Urea and creatinine can rise in pre-eclampsia, reflecting renal involvement.
- Urate. Increased levels of uric acid are often an early finding in pre-eclampsia.
- Clotting screen. This is rarely abnormal without a concomitant fall in platelets.
- Liver function tests (LFTs). The transaminases may be increased in pre-eclampsia. This is an important sign of HELLP syndrome (haemolysis, elevated liver enzymes and low platelets) (see below) but can occur in the absence of haemolysis and low platelets. Note that alkaline phosphatase is produced by the liver and placenta, so is normally raised in pregnancy.
- Midstream urine for culture and sensitivity. Infection can cause proteinuria, and invalidates protein quantification.
- 24-hour urinary protein. This is important in defining the disease, with greater than 300 mg in 24 hours being significant.
- Ultrasound scan of the fetus for biometry, liquor volume and umbilical artery Doppler.

The signs and symptoms of pre-eclampsia can develop at different times and at different rates in individual women. It is best thought of as a syndrome where any of the following may occur:

- New onset hypertension (>140/90 is usually used, as this reflects maternal and fetal morbidity better than an incremental rise). Blood pressure should be measured sitting, and the Korotkoff V sound (disappearance of sound) should be used as opposed to Korotkoff IV (muffling). It should also be noted that electronic blood pressure devices tend to under-measure blood pressure in pre-eclampsia and measurement with an anodyne device should always be taken once.

- Proteinuria of + or more.
- Symptoms of headache/epigastric pain/visual disturbance.
- Evidence of organ dysfunction (raised urea/creatinine/urates/liver function tests or low platelets).

When two out of any of the above are present, pre-eclampsia is likely to be present. Review at hospital should be arranged when any two are present, and should be considered for any single finding. A recent British Medical Journal article provides an excellent framework for the management of pre-eclampsia when in a community setting.[9]

Having confirmed the diagnosis, management principally depends on the severity of the condition and the gestation. Diagnosis can be difficult when there is renal disease with hypertension predating the pre-eclampsia.

At early gestations (under 34 weeks), it may be valuable to prolong the pregnancy if possible, certainly to allow administration of steroids. Maternal and fetal surveillance is important, and in moderate or severe pre-eclampsia this must be undertaken in hospital:

- 4–6-hourly blood pressure readings
- Daily urinalysis
- Blood tests are usually repeated every 72 hours
- Daily cardiotocograph (CTG).

There is limited value in repeating the 24-hour urine collection once significant proteinuria has been established, as this rarely guides the need for delivery. At earlier gestations delivery is more commonly undertaken for fetal reasons. Repeated umbilical artery Doppler assessments on the fetus may be required once or twice weekly, with biometry undertaken every 2 weeks. A daily CTG is usually undertaken. Escalation in blood pressure control, or symptoms of impending eclampsia are other reasons for delivery.

At later gestations the balance of risk tends to favour delivery. Unless the fetus is acutely unwell or with severe growth restriction and significantly abnormal umbilical artery Doppler, this can often be achieved by induction of labour.

Investigation after delivery

These women require follow-up to ensure their blood pressure returns to normal and the proteinuria disappears. This may take several weeks. If the blood pressure remains elevated, investigation should be considered (as for chronic hypertension). If the proteinuria does not resolve by 3 months postpartum, it should be quantified having excluded infection. If significant, and especially if more than 1 g in 24 hours, consideration should be given to referral to a nephrologist for investigation.

Women with severe early onset disease should be investigated for antiphospholipid syndrome postnatally (see Ch. 4, Haematology).

HELLP syndrome

This is a severe variant of pre-eclampsia characterised by haemolysis, elevated liver enzymes and low platelets (less than 100 000/mm^3). Haemolysis is usually evident on a blood film, and lactate dehydrogenase will be elevated.[10]

RENAL DISEASE

Pregnancy has profound effects on the kidney and results of investigations must be interpreted in the context of these physiological changes (see Box 5.5). These are most notably:

- Increased renal blood flow of 80%, with a concomitant increase in glomerular filtration rate of 50%. As a consequence, serum urea and creatinine fall.
- Dilatation of the urinary collecting system more pronounced on the right.
- Increased fluid retention resulting in oedema in 80% of pregnant women by term.
- Increased protein excretion.

Box 5.5 Normal values in pregnancy related to changes in renal function	
Creatinine clearance	120–160 ml/min
Protein excretion	< 0.3 g in 24 hours
Sodium	Same as non-pregnant
Potassium	Same as non-pregnant
Urate	Gestation specific with fall in first trimester and rise to above non-pregnant range in late pregnancy. Mean 269 micromol/l at 38 weeks
Urea	2.0–4.5 mmol/l
Creatinine	25–75 micromol/l

Infection

Asymptomatic bacteriuria is relatively common in pregnancy and if untreated may progress to symptomatic infection. Thus all women should have a midstream specimen of urine (MSU) sent for culture and sensitivity at the start of pregnancy. Urinalysis alone is not sufficiently sensitive to use as a screening test.

Interpretation of the MSU is important. Bacteriuria is only considered significant if the colony count exceeds 100 000 per ml. Mixed culture often results from contamination and should prompt repeat testing. The woman should be advised of appropriate technique in collecting the sample, so minimising the risk of contamination.

Symptoms of cystitis, most notably dysuria (frequency is common in pregnancy), should prompt urine culture and sensitivity. Cystitis should be distinguished from acute pyelonephritis that signifies ascent of the infection to one or both kidneys. The woman with lower urinary tract infection can be treated with antibiotics and increased fluid as an outpatient. The GP should consider a 5–7 day course of antibiotics. A test of cure should be undertaken 7–14 days after completion of the course. In the woman prone to recurrent urinary tract infections with E. coli, a glass of cranberry juice a day can help to prevent recurrence. A chemical in cranberries prevents pathogenic E. coli from adhering to the bladder wall.

The woman with pyelonephritis is usually systemically unwell with pyrexia, rigors and loin or abdominal pain. In this case admission to hospital is required and the following investigations should be undertaken:

- FBC. The white cell count may be raised with a neutrophilia.
- Urea, creatinine and electrolytes. There may be dehydration as a consequence of vomiting and insensible losses (higher with pyrexia), with electrolyte imbalance. If severely affected there may be renal impairment. Regular assessment is necessary (usually daily in the acute phase).
- Blood cultures. These should be undertaken if pyrexial.
- Ultrasound of kidneys and renal tract. This is important if there is not a prompt response to intravenous antibiotics as there may be hydronephrosis, congenital abnormalities or calculi predisposing to the infection.

Chronic renal disease: primary glomerular diseases

Primary glomerular diseases are dealt with as a group here as in general it is not the specific disease that determines the impact upon pregnancy, but rather the presence or absence of risk factors associated with nephropathy at booking. The most influential factors for prognosis are:

- Nephrotic range proteinuria (greater than 3.5 g in 24 hours)
- Hypertension
- Impaired renal function.

Thus women known to have a primary glomerular disease should ideally have received pre-conception counselling based on the above factors. These risk factors have additive effects, and some women experience a non-reversible worsening of renal function during pregnancy.

During pregnancy protein excretion usually increases, but often returns to pre-pregnant levels after delivery. The main difficulty this poses to the clinician is determining whether pre-eclampsia is present. These women are already at increased risk of developing this complication in their pregnancy. Clinical features including escalation of hypertension and symptoms of pre-eclampsia, together with the regular monitoring outlined below, will help to detect pre-eclampsia.

Poorly controlled hypertension at booking is an important prognostic factor, and early control is essential.

The degree of impaired renal function is categorised by the serum creatinine and creatinine clearance. In general, renal impairment can be classified as:

- Mild   (serum creatinine < 125 micromol/l)
- Moderate   (serum creatinine 125–250 micromol/l)
- Severe   (serum creatinine > 250 micromol/l).[11]

During pregnancy it is important to regularly undertake:

- Full blood count. Chronic disease may cause a normochromic normocytic anaemia that does not respond to iron therapy. In pre-eclampsia the platelets may fall.
- Serum urea and creatinine.
- Creatinine clearance and protein excretion.
- Liver function tests. These may become deranged with pre-eclampsia.
- MSU.
- Fetal biometry and umbilical artery Doppler, because of an increased risk of growth restriction.

Renal transplant recipients

More women are now regaining fertility after transplantation. Ideally they should wait for 2 years after the transplant before conceiving. Assessment is similar to that outlined above. Calcium status should also be checked. An additional complication to be aware of is graft rejection and immunosuppressant drug toxicity. Management requires expertise from nephrologists.

Nephrolithiasis

Nephrolithiasis (renal stones) usually pre-dates the pregnancy. The main concerns are renal colic and urinary tract infection. Renal colic results from obstruction of the renal pelvis or ureter, and pain

may mimic uterine contractions. It is, however, usually unilateral and closer to the loin, radiating down the flank. Haematuria is often (though not invariably) present.

Investigation should include:

- Urinalysis. Haematuria is often present.
- Midstream urine for culture and sensitivity.
- FBC. White cell count (WCC) may be raised if infection is present.
- Urea, creatinine and electrolytes.
- Renal ultrasound as a first line imaging modality:
  - Minimally invasive
  - No contrast media required
  - Can confuse renal tract dilatation of pregnancy with obstruction
  - Difficult to visualise ureters.

If the clinical suspicion is high despite an apparently normal ultrasound, other investigations should be considered following discussion with an urologist.

Diabetic nephropathy

See diabetes.

Acute renal failure

This is rare and may result from sepsis, blood loss, pre-eclampsia and ureteric damage or obstruction.

Investigations will be geared to the clinical picture.

CARDIAC DISEASE

Pregnancy is associated with an increase in cardiac output of approximately 40%, and a decrease in peripheral vascular resistance. Thus there are significant alterations in the circulation in pregnancy that those with heart disease may struggle to withstand.

Many symptoms and signs of heart disease can be found in normal pregnancy. For example, breathlessness is often physiological. More telling is whether this symptom pre-dated the pregnancy. Syncope (a faint) is also encountered in healthy pregnancies, but may signify significant cardiac disease. Oedema is found in 80% of pregnant women. Ejection systolic murmurs are common, and relate to increased blood flow across the heart valves. Various features of murmurs mean they are more likely to indicate pathology, such as pansystolic murmurs. However, it is subtle features such as this that require an experienced 'ear', and cardiologists cannot be expected to see all women in pregnancy with a murmur. Selective auscultation is likely to be more productive. Young Caucasian women without a history of a congenital cardiac defect, and without symptoms, are unlikely to have significant heart disease and do not require routine auscultation of the heart at booking. However, certain women are at higher risk of acquired heart disease, such as immigrants from areas where rheumatic heart disease is prevalent. There should be a low threshold for investigating these women with symptoms or signs that in other situations might be attributed to normal pregnancy.

Congenital heart disease

Most women with congenital cardiac anomalies will know of this before embarking on pregnancy, and many will have undergone surgical correction. However, as the latest Confidential Enquiry into Maternal and Child Health (CEMACH) report[12] points out, these women are still at risk from fluctuations in circulating volume as surgical correction of their lesions is often of necessity incomplete. Although most will tolerate pregnancy well, clinicians must be alert to symptoms and signs of decompensation, and refer appropriately.

Symptoms of worsening heart disease include:

- increasing breathlessness (especially at night)
- decreasing exercise tolerance
- episodes of palpitations
- chest pain
- worsening oedema.

Echocardiography is the investigation of choice for structural heart disease.

Women at risk of developing pulmonary hypertension from their congenital cardiac disease should have echocardiography repeated during pregnancy even if it was normal before pregnancy. Eisenmenger's syndrome (usually an atrial septal defect or ventricular septal defect with pulmonary hypertension and a reversed shunt across the defect, i.e. from right to left) has a 30–50% maternal mortality.

It should be remembered that congenital cardiac malformations are more common in the baby born to an affected mother. Thus a fetal echocardiogram should be undertaken.

Acquired heart disease

Rheumatic heart disease is the principal acquired heart disease worldwide, and most commonly is seen as mitral stenosis. This can be dangerous in pregnancy. Thus, women who were brought up in areas of high prevalence (Asian sub-continent, Africa, some parts of the Middle East and Far East) should be carefully questioned regarding symptoms of heart disease, and signs should be sought, heart sounds auscultated and echocardiography undertaken readily.

Ischaemic heart disease is reported in the CEMACH report,[12] and reflects the fact that older women are embarking on pregnancy. Risk factors should be taken note of: smoking, hypertension, obesity and family history. Diabetes is also a risk factor. Coronary artery dissection can cause myocardial infarction, and a low threshold for angiography should be maintained if myocardial infarction in pregnancy occurs. Myocardial infarction is diagnosed on the basis of electrocardiogram changes together with a raised serum troponin I level (released by damaged myocardium).

Dissecting aortic aneurysm is rare but must be considered in women presenting with chest pain in pregnancy. Often the symptoms are initially attributed to a pulmonary embolism. A widened aorta may be seen on chest X-ray. Magnetic resonance imaging can be used for diagnosis. If confirmed, Marfan's syndrome, an autosomal dominant condition, should be considered.

Cardiomyopathy may present with signs of heart failure, and echocardiography is used to make the diagnosis. This may present postpartum and is usually in older mothers.

Arrhythmias are abnormal rhythms of the heart that commonly present with palpitations and dizziness. A sinus tachycardia is not uncommon in normal pregnancy but investigation should include thyroid function tests and electrocardiogram. An infective aetiology should also be considered.

If intermittent symptoms occur suggestive of a supraventricular tachycardia, a 24-hour cardiac tape should be requested. Again, thyroid function tests should be done to exclude thyrotoxicosis.

EPILEPSY

Epilepsy takes various forms, but is usually idiopathic (no identifiable cause). Most women have already had a diagnosis made. Seizures may increase in pregnancy, and this can be associated with nausea and vomiting in early pregnancy, poor compliance due to fears of teratogenesis, and reduced drug levels due to the increased plasma volume.

Monitoring anticonvulsant levels is not necessary unless seizures increase in frequency or poor compliance is suspected.[13]

Information about contraception and pregnancy should be given to all women of childbearing age with epilepsy. Folic acid 5 mg daily should be started before conception as there is an increased risk of neural tube defects. All women should be offered serum alpha-fetoprotein screening for neural tube defects around 16 weeks' gestation, and detailed ultrasound at 20–22 weeks with particular emphasis on looking at the spine, heart and face. Even if there is no apparent anomaly, fetuses can be affected with an anti-epileptic drug syndrome causing various dysmorphic features, and pregnant women need to be informed of this. The risk is higher in women taking more than one medication. Sodium valproate is most implicated, but this has to be balanced against the fact that this is the most suitable drug for many women with generalised seizures.

If a woman presents in pregnancy with a seizure for the first time, it is important to get a witnessed account of the event if possible. The following investigations should be considered:

- Blood pressure and urinalysis (possible eclampsia)
- FBC, clotting screen, urea and electrolytes (U&E), LFT, urate
- Serum calcium
- Blood glucose
- CT or MRI of brain
- Electroencephalogram (EEG).

In general it is safe for women on anti-epileptic drugs to breast feed, but where doubt exists, information is available in the British National Formulary.[14] This also lists telephone numbers for regional medicine information services.

RESPIRATORY DISEASE

There is a physiological hyperventilation in pregnancy, and some women are aware of breathlessness related to this. Breathlessness should not be assumed to be physiological; further investigation may be warranted.

Asthma

Asthma is the commonest respiratory disease encountered in pregnancy, and is generally managed in the same way as outside of pregnancy. Wheeze is a characteristic feature. The peak expiratory flow rate (PEFR) is an easy test to perform, and usually shows a characteristic daytime variance, and improves in response to an inhaled beta sympathomimetic drug. The most important advice to women is to continue their regular inhalers. If a short course of oral steroids is required, women can be reassured that this is safe for the fetus.

If asthma is severe, requiring hospital admission, investigation should include PEFR and oxygen saturation. If life-threatening features are present, arterial blood gases should be obtained. A chest X-ray is required if pneumothorax or infection are suspected, or there is a failure of response to treatment.

Pneumonia

Pneumonia in pregnancy may be bacterial or viral. The features are similar to outside of pregnancy, namely breathlessness, chest pain and fever. Investigation should include:

- FBC
- Chest X-ray
- Sputum culture
- Arterial blood gases.

Varicella-zoster pneumonia is a complication of chickenpox and of particular concern in pregnancy as it tends to be more severe.

Tuberculosis

Tuberculosis is increasing in the UK and is more common amongst Asian and African immigrants. Cough, sometimes with haemoptysis, and weight loss are characteristic. Again chest X-ray should be performed, and sputum examined for acid-fast bacilli. Consideration should be given to the possibility of co-infection with HIV.

Cystic fibrosis

Women with *cystic fibrosis* are now surviving into adulthood, and experiencing pregnancy. This is an autosomal recessive condition, and offspring will inevitably be carriers. It is important to offer screening of the partner in terms of assessing risk to the offspring. Pregnancy is well tolerated by most mothers, and should be managed jointly with a cystic fibrosis team. The diabetologist may also be involved as many of these women have diabetes as a result of pancreatic insufficiency. The chronic lung infection results in reduced forced expiratory volume in 1 second (FEV_1), and severity can be assessed by spirometry. Hypoxaemia increases the risk, as does pulmonary hypertension. Regular sputum samples should guide antibiotic treatment. Regular biometry should be undertaken on the fetus as there is an increased risk of growth restriction.

CONNECTIVE TISSUE DISEASE

Inflammatory arthritides

These are divided into seropositive and seronegative arthritides. The commonest seropositive arthritis is rheumatoid arthritis. This is an autoimmune disorder affecting the synovial joints, with progressive joint damage. All women with arthritides should be referred for consultant obstetric care, as there are implications for the management of joint pain, mobility and drug treatment. In some seropositive arthritides, the autoimmune component may have consequences for the pregnancy and early referral is needed.

Approximately 40% of women with rheumatoid arthritis will have antibodies, such as Ro or anti-La. These antibodies can cross the placenta and destroy the Purkinje fibres of the developing fetal heart, leading to congenital heart block in 35–40% of fetuses in positive mothers. This occurs between 16 and 26 weeks. In anti-Ro positive mothers, weekly auscultation of the fetal heart to detect missed beats (usually the first sign) or bradycardia is needed. A word of caution in interpretation of investigations is that the erythrocyte sedimentation rate, a marker of inflammatory activity, is not useful in pregnancy as it is normally raised. The C-reactive protein is not affected by pregnancy and can be used to determine inflammatory states.

Systemic lupus erythematosus (SLE)

This is an autoimmune connective tissue disease that manifests in various ways, most commonly with arthritis. There can also be skin, renal and neurological manifestations. The disease is characterised by periods of activity (flare) and remission. The diagnosis has again usually been established before pregnancy, and pre-pregnancy counselling is important. The diagnosis is made on the basis of clinical features together with serological markers, namely certain autoantibodies. The commonest of these is anti-nuclear antibody (ANA), but this can be found in women without SLE. More specific is anti-double stranded DNA antibody (anti-DNA), and this is useful to measure in assessing lupus flare.[15] Anti-Ro, anti-La and antiphospholipid antibodies are important to measure as these increase the risk to the pregnancy (see above).

Management should be in a multidisciplinary setting. Periods of disease activity can be difficult to diagnose. Renal involvement is easily confused with pre-eclampsia, but the finding of a rise in anti-DNA antibody titre, and a fall in complement levels, can help point towards the flare.[15]

The presence of antiphospholipid antibodies can occur without SLE but confers an increased risk of fetal loss (see Ch. 4). Anti-Ro and anti-La antibodies can cause neonatal lupus syndromes by crossing the placenta. This can manifest as skin lesions or congenital heart block.[16]

Medications used in SLE include cytotoxic agents such as cyclophosphamide. Pre-pregnancy counselling enables a discussion on which medications are safe to use both in pregnancy and when breast feeding.

LIVER DISEASE

It is useful to remember that pregnancy results in a normal increase in alkaline phosphatase as this is produced by the placenta. The transaminases alanine aminotransferase (ALT) and aspartate aminotransferase (AST) fall slightly as pregnancy progresses, and the bilirubin level is unchanged.

Intrahepatic cholestasis of pregnancy

This is a condition occurring in the second half of pregnancy, where bile produced by the liver accumulates in the blood. It is characterised clinically by pruritis, initially of the extremities but later generalised, in the absence of a rash. Excoriations may be present from scratching. Jaundice may occur. A history of a rash predating the pruritis is probably due to a different pathology.

Biochemical changes are used to confirm the diagnosis. The most sensitive finding is a raised serum bile acid concentration, often combined with a rise in the transaminases. If the transaminases are normal, the bile acids must be checked as a raised concentration may be the sole biochemical finding. Where tests are normal but symptoms persist, blood tests should be repeated after a week.

The diagnosis relies on exclusion of other causes of elevated liver enzymes. The following additional tests should be considered:

- Clotting screen. Cholestasis can impair absorption of fat-soluble vitamins, e.g. vitamin K needed for synthesis of clotting factors.
- U&E, urate. These should be undertaken if there is clinical suspicion of pre-eclampsia.
- Serology for hepatitis A, B, C, Epstein–Barr virus and cytomegalovirus.
- Ultrasound scan of liver and gall bladder.
- Autoantibodies in case of rare diseases such as primary biliary cirrhosis.

The chief concern relates to the fetus, with an increased risk of preterm delivery, intrapartum fetal compromise, meconium staining of the liquor, and fetal death.[17] In view of these concerns it is advocated that increased fetal surveillance be undertaken, although fetal compromise remains unpredictable. Usually a combination of fort-

nightly growth scans with liquor volume and umbilical artery Doppler, and twice weekly CTGs, are undertaken, although this must be individualised depending on the gestation and other risk factors. LFTs are usually monitored weekly if on treatment. Delivery is usually planned at around 37 weeks.

The condition resolves after delivery. If LFTs do not quickly return to normal, an alternative diagnosis should be considered. The combined oral contraceptive pill should be avoided. The recurrence risk may be as high as 90%, and women should thus be readily tested if symptomatic in a future pregnancy.

Key Practice Points

- Midwives should ensure they are familiar with the commoner pre-existing medical conditions that are seen in pregnancy.
- Most conditions require multidisciplinary input with at least an obstetrician and physician.
- Blood pressure and urinalysis are essential in early pregnancy; an MSU should also be sent for culture and sensitivity.
- Test results should be interpreted in the context of pregnancy; it is important to be aware of differences from the non-pregnant state.

References

1. Umpierrez GE, Latif, KA, Murphy MB, et al. Thyroid dysfunction in patients With Type 1 diabetes: a longitudinal study. Diabetes Care 2003; 26(4):1181–1185.
2. Kyne-Grzebalski D, Wood L, Marshall S M, Taylor R. Episodic hyperglycaemia in pregnant women with well-controlled Type 1 diabetes mellitus: a major potential factor underlying macrosomia. Diabetic Medicine 1999; 16(8):702.
3. Kamalakannan D, Baskar V, Barton D M, Abdu TAM. Diabetic ketoacidosis in pregnancy. Postgrad Med J 2003; 79:454–457.
4. National Institute for Clinical Excellence. Antenatal care: routine care for the healthy pregnant woman. London: RCOG Press; 2003. Online. Available: www.nice.org.uk/page.aspx?o=89893

5. Pop VJ, Kuijpens JL, van Bar AL, Verker G, van Son MM. Low maternal free thyroxine concentrations during early pregnancy are associated with impaired psychomotor development in infancy. Clinical Endocrinology 1999; 50:149–155.

6. Lazarus JH, Kokandi A. Thyroid disease in relation to pregnancy: a decade of change. Clinical Endocrinology 2000; 53(3):265–278.

7. Sibai BM. Chronic hypertension in pregnancy. Obstetrics & Gynaecology 2002; 100(2):369–377.

8. Redman CWG, Sacks GP, Sargent IL. Preeclampsia: an excessive maternal inflammatory response to pregnancy. Am J Obstet Gynecol 1999; 180:499–506.

9. Milne F, Redman C, Walker J, et al. The pre-eclampsia community guideline (PRECOG): how to screen for and detect onset of pre-eclampsia in the community. BMJ Mar 2005; 330:576–580.

10. Witlin AG, Sibai BM. HELLP syndrome. Hospital Physician 1999; 49:40–45.

11. Davison J, Baylis C. Renal disease. In: de Swiet M, ed. Medical disorders in obstetric practice. 3rd edn. Oxford: Blackwell Science; 1995:226–305.

12. CEMACH, Lewis G, ed. Why mothers die 2000–2002. The sixth report of the Confidential Enquiries into Maternal Deaths in the UK. London: RCOG Press; 2004 Online. Available: www.cemach.org.uk/publications/WMD 2000-2002/content.htm.

13. National Institute for Clinical Excellence. The epilepsies: the diagnosis and management of the epilepsies in adults and children in primary and secondary care. London: National Institute for Clinical Excellence; 2004.

14. British National Formulary No. 49. London: British Medical Association and Royal Pharmaceutical Society of Great Britain; 2005.

15. Mok C, Wong RWS. Pregnancy in systemic lupus erythematosus. Postgrad Med J 2001; 77:157–165.

16. Nelson-Piercy C. Handbook of obstetric medicine. Oxford: Isis Medical Media; 1997.

17. Mullaly BA, Hansen WF. Intrahepatic cholestasis of pregnancy: review of the literature. Obstetrical & Gynecological Survey 2002; 57(1):47–52.

6

Infections in pregnancy

William Martin, Ellen Knox

INTRODUCTION

Any infection may develop in pregnancy but few affect the pregnancy adversely. Pregnancy does not usually increase the severity of an infection; however, due to a relatively immunocompromised state, secondary to the physiological changes of pregnancy, certain maternal infections, such as urinary tract infections and pneumonia, are more likely to occur.

Fetal or neonatal infections may be acquired in utero (congenital by transplacental spread); at time of delivery (intrapartum by exposure to vaginal/cervical secretions, maternal blood or faeces); or neonatally (postpartum from breast feeding, direct contact or by respiratory route).

Any adverse effect on the fetus may be a teratogenic effect (e.g. rubella, toxoplasmosis) or be caused indirectly (e.g. cytomegalovirus, chicken pox). The timing of infection is important in determining the outcome of an infection. First trimester infection leads to structural abnormalities more often than later infections. Infection may lead to growth restriction (often symmetrical) and preterm delivery with adverse sequelae accruing as a result.

Although potential fetal effects may be well established, it may be difficult to identify a woman who has been infected. Many viral infections with potential for severe fetal effects will pass unrecognised through lack of symptoms—often the pregnant woman will show no ill effects or at most have non-specific viral symptoms. Even if the mother is proven to have had infection, the fetus may not become infected; and even if infected, the fetal outcome is often uncertain and difficult to predict varying from none to profound. These factors make the investigation and management of such pregnancies very difficult.

This chapter will discuss some of the various viral, bacterial and parasytic infections that can adversely affect pregnancy. Some of the infections to be discussed are subject to routine antenatal screening (e.g. asymptomatic bacteriuria, hepatitis B and HIV). Others are potential future targets for routine screening, such as group B streptococcal and chlamydial infections. The common symptoms and presentation of the infections in pregnancy are discussed. The effects of the infections both on the mother and fetus/neonate are considered along with diagnostic procedures and management strategies.

BACTERIAL INFECTIONS

Group B *streptococcus* (GBS)

This infection has been the subject of much concern recently. Although not currently the subject of routine antenatal screening, it may soon be, however current evidence does not support this. It is often an incidental finding on vaginal swabs or urine culture performed for other indications. Recent guidance from the Royal College of Obstetricians and Gynaecologists (RCOG) has provided a useful guideline on the management of women known to carry GBS.[1]

Maternal

The organism is a normal commensal found in up to 20% of women at any one time during pregnancy. GBS may lead to puerperal sepsis and formerly was considered a risk factor for preterm delivery. Whether GBS is associated with preterm labour is currently debatable, previous associations are probably coincidental. Chorioamnionitis and endometritis have both been associated with GBS. The major significance of this bacterial infection is its potential for causing severe illness in the newborn.

Group B streptococcus (GBS) may best be identified by low vaginal and rectal swabs as the gastrointestinal tract is its primary reservoir. Treatment antenatally should only be given for GBS found on midstream specimen of urine (MSU). Antepartum antibiotic treatment is otherwise ineffective and may increase the presence of other resistant pathogenic bacteria.

Fetal and neonatal

There are probably no fetal effects of GBS in isolation. In the first week of life up to 12% of neonates will be colonised, this figure rising to 70% of babies born to colonised mothers. The factors that influence colonisation include the degree of maternal colonisation, cervical carriage and GBS in maternal urine.

GBS can cause invasive neonatal disease leading to sepsis, pneumonia and meningitis. In the 1970s the mortality was over 50% in such cases. This has reduced dramatically in recent years. In the UK the incidence of invasive disease is around 1 in 1000 live births. The invasive disease may be of early (80% of cases) or late onset. The former has a median onset of 20 hours and is due to vertical transmission, the latter occurs after 7 days with half of cases due to vertical transmission, the rest due to nosocomial spread from infants, staff and other adults.

The risk factors for early onset GBS are shown in Box 6.1.

Box 6.1   Risk factors for early onset group B Streptococcal infection

Pre-pregnancy
- Age <20 years
- African–American descent
- Australian Aboriginal descent
- Previously affected baby

Antepartum
- GBS bacteriuria in pregnancy
- Heavy colonisation
- Low levels anti-GBS capsular antibodies
- Prelabour rupture membranes

Intrapartum
- Preterm delivery
- Pyrexia >38°C
- Ruptured membranes >18 hours

The prevention of neonatal disease can be achieved through the use of intrapartum antibiotics, a recent Cochrane review reached this conclusion although randomised controlled trials are lacking.[2]

The antibiotic of choice is penicillin. The narrow spectrum of this antibiotic is effective against GBS but should avoid resistance developing for other bacteria. Treatment is initially 3 g benzylpenicillin intravenously (ideally 4 hours prior to delivery) followed by 1.5 g intravenously every 4 hours. In the penicillin allergic, clindamycin (900 mg intravenously 8 hourly) is an appropriate alternative.

Women who should receive intrapartum prophylaxis are those with:

- a previously affected baby
- GBS as an incidental finding on vaginal swabbing
- GBS isolated from a specimen of urine.

As mentioned, screening is not currently recommended. There are various strategies used to screen for GBS and these result in varying proportions of pregnant mothers receiving antibiotic prophylaxis, many of whom are either notcolonised or are at low risk of neonatal GBS infection.

There are disadvantages of intrapartum prophylaxis. It may lead to treatment of unaffected women who may get adverse reactions to penicillin. One in 100 000 will die through anaphylaxis and a further 1:10 000 will suffer minor sequelae. Resistance is an ever-present concern and has been described. The routine use of antibiotics intravenously leads to medicalisation of labour; indeed, after counselling women may decline treatment because of this. The mother and neonate may have to spend 48 hours in hospital for observation if prophylaxis was inadequate. This again is over-medicalisation, preventing early discharge from hospital.

Prophylaxis may not prevent neonatal infection. The amount of colonisation is reduced but only temporarily and thus does not protect against late onset GBS infection which can lead to serious neonatal morbidity and mortality.

The ability to target treatment may be improved if rapid testing techniques currently being developed prove effective.

Key Practice Points

- There is no current evidence to recommend universal screening.
- Intrapartum antibiotic prophylaxis reduces early onset neonatal infection.
- High-risk groups (Box 6.1) should be offered antibiotic prophylaxis in labour.
- Neonatal swabs should be taken at delivery and the baby observed for 24 hours. Alert the paediatric team to the mother's GBS status and risk factors.
- On discharge the community midwifery team and GP should be specifically informed.

Asymptomatic bacteriuria

This is defined as the presence of >10^5 bacteria/ml of a midstream specimen of urine (MSU) in the absence of symptoms such as dysuria and haematuria. In pregnancy the other classic symptoms of urinary tract infection (UTI), frequency and urgency, are unreliable. The most commonly utilised test is the MSU; however, the use of dipstick testing to include protein, blood, leucocyte esterase (an enzyme from neutrophils indicating pyuria) and nitrites (indicative of bacterial activity) have been used with varying results. The dipstick may provide an apparent cost saving over an MSU but there are drawbacks, including the wide variation in sensitivity and specificity. The significance of finding asymptomatic bacteriuria is its association with the later development of pyelonephritis, itself associated with premature labour and intrauterine growth restriction.

Screening is currently recommended by the National Screening Committee (NSC) as identification and treatment of asymptomatic bacteriuria reduces preterm birth.[3]

Maternal

Six percent of women will develop asymptomatic bacteriuria. Of those, 17% will develop pyelonephritis.

Fetal and neonatal

Older data suggested an association between bacteriuria and preterm labour. In addition, it seemed that antibiotic treatment reduced the risk.[4] The association between pyelonephritis and preterm delivery was apparent in early studies; however, this does not appear to be seen in more modern studies. This may be because prompt treatment of infection prevents preterm labour progressing to preterm birth. There does not appear to be a significant association between asymptomatic bacteriuria and preterm birth unless pyelonephritis supervenes.

Key Practice Points

- Currently all women should be screened for asymptomatic bacteriuria at booking.
- Antibiotic treatment for 5–7 days is indicated.

Bacterial vaginosis

Within the vagina, lactobacilli are the predominant species with low levels of anaerobic bacteria present under normal conditions. If the vaginal pH increases— at menstruation or after candidal infections—overgrowth of these anaerobic bacteria occur with the concomitant decrease in the natural lactobacilli within the vagina. This disturbance in the normal flora results in an increase in pH above 4.5, which permits an increase in anaerobic bacteria leading to clinical bacterial vaginosis (BV). The initiating event is unknown. The condition is associated with poor pregnancy outcome but is amenable, at least temporarily, to antibiotic therapy. Whether treatment reduces the associated pregnancy risks is uncertain. Bacterial vaginosis is a co-factor for sexually transmitted infections (STIs), including human immunodeficiency virus (HIV) and trichomonal infection.

It is the commonest cause of non-physiological vaginal discharge with rates of up to 20% in unselected populations. In 50% of women the condition is asymptomatic. Diagnosis can be made from the presence of three out of four of Amsel's criteria (see Box 6.2). In addition, Gram staining is a reliable method of diagnosis.

The bacteria involved include *Gardenerella vaginalis, Mobiluncus, Bacteriodes, Mycoplasma hominis,*

Box 6.2 Amsel's criteria for the clinical diagnosis of bacterial vaginosis

- Thin, homogeneous, white/yellow discharge
- Clue cells on microscopy (wet film)
- pH >4.5
- Characteristic fishy odour on addition of 10% potassium hydroxide to vaginal fluid.

Ureaplasma urealyticum. The presence of any of these alone, however, is not sufficient for the diagnosis of BV to be made. In particular the *G. vaginalis* may be found in up to 50% of healthy women without BV.

Maternal

There are few maternal complications; however, BV has been associated with endometritis. It has also been shown to be related to second trimester pregnancy loss (5-fold increase), preterm premature rupture of the membranes (PPROM) (7-fold increase) and preterm birth (5-fold increase).[5] No convincing evidence of first trimester loss has been found.

Fetal and neonatal

There are several influences that BV may have on the fetus and neonate. Bacterial vaginosis has been associated with preterm labour, PPROM and chorioamnionitis. Recent evidence shows the presence of pro-inflammatory cytokines interleukin (IL)-1, IL-6 and tumour necrosis factor α (TNFα) in samples from the amniotic fluid and from the lower genital tract in pregnancies affected by BV. These factors are of fetal origin, indicative of a fetal systemic inflammatory response syndrome. Studies have related the development of periventricular leucomalacia and cerebral palsy (CP) in preterm infants to these cytokines which may indicate a link between infection with BV and CP.[6]

Current recommendations from the Centers for Disease Control and Prevention in the USA are that in high risk pregnancies where there has either been a previous preterm birth with or without associated BV or there is evidence of other STIs, screening for BV should be undertaken and treated as appropriate (see below). For unselected pregnancies the picture is less clear. Studies have often screened late in pregnancy when the opportunity to prevent preterm birth has been missed. There is currently insufficient evidence to recommend screening an unselected population.

Metronidazole (400 mg twice daily for 5 days) is effective against BV but is only active against anaerobes, not other species associated with BV such as *G. vaginalis*. Clindamycin is an appropriate alternative. Treatment failure is common and may relate to persistence of *G. vaginalis*.

> **Key Practice Points**
>
> - BV is associated with poor pregnancy outcome.
> - Screening for BV is not currently recommended.
> - However, those with previous BV and previous premature delivery should be screened at booking.
> - Symptomatic confirmed infection should be treated.
> - Metronidazole or clindamycin are appropriate treatments.

VIRAL INFECTIONS

Viral infections can have profound and devastating effects on the fetus, often with little evidence of clinical infection in the mother. Immunity may have been conferred, either through vaccination (e.g. rubella) or through childhood contact (e.g. chicken pox (varicella/zoster). The ability to predict outcome accurately relies on history of previous childhood infection, serological testing, invasive testing (amniocentesis, fetal blood sampling) and serial ultrasound scanning. Even with these tests prognosis may be difficult/impossible to predict. This causes a great deal of anxiety for the parents for whom the possible outcome of the pregnancy may vary from no/little effect to the birth of a potentially severely and profoundly handicapped child.

In general, the timing of the infection has a bearing on outcome with infection in the first trimester having greater significance than later infections. It must be borne in mind that maternal infection does not equal fetal infection. In turn, fetal infection does not mean that the fetus will be affected. It is advisable to consult with a microbiologist/virologist and patients at risk should be referred to a centre with expertise in fetal medicine, as management of these infections is difficult.

Rubella

Rubella is a ribonucleic acid (RNA) virus spread through respiratory droplets or by transmission in utero, with potentially devastating effects. In many, clinical symptoms are lacking but if present include general malaise, fever and a maculopapular pink/red rash that begins on the forehead and then spreads to the trunk and limbs and usually lasts for 3 days. Conjunctivitis and lymphadenopathy (postauricular and suboccipital) are common. Serious sequelae are not common.

Maternal

Complications are rare but can include pneumonia, arthralgia, encephalitis and thrombocytopenia leading to haemorrhagic complications.

Diagnosis is usually possible on clinical grounds but can be confirmed using culture of urine, nasopharyngeal swabs and cerebrospinal fluid analysis. Serological testing is the most useful available test. It is recommended that any pregnant woman developing a non-vesicular rash should be investigated for rubella (and parvovirus B19) irrespective of her previous tests. Similarly, if a woman has been in contact (face-to-face or in the same room for 15 minutes) with a person with a non-vesicular rash, investigations for rubella (and parvovirus B19) should be performed.

Fetal infection may be diagnosed using fetal blood sampling. The presence of IgM to rubella can only be evidence of fetal infection as the IgM molecule is too large to cross the placenta. However, this may not be present until after 19 weeks' gestation. Polymerase chain reaction (PCR) for viral RNA can also be used with amniotic fluid

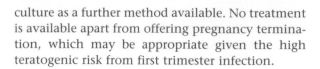

culture as a further method available. No treatment is available apart from offering pregnancy termination, which may be appropriate given the high teratogenic risk from first trimester infection.

Fetal and neonatal

The major significance of rubella in pregnancy is its potential for adverse fetal effects. It is for this reason that rubella immunisation is offered to all children (previously girls in the early teens). Any patient of child bearing age who is planning a pregnancy should be checked for immunity, thus patients attending fertility clinics and for pre-pregnancy counselling should be tested routinely. Rubella immunity is part of the routine antenatal screening programme in early pregnancy. If found to be non-immune, the patient should be advised to avoid known contacts and anyone with a non-vesicular rash. Postnatal immunisation should be carried out using the triple vaccine for measles mumps and rubella (MMR) (single rubella vaccine is no longer available). Antepartum vaccination is not used as there is a theoretical risk of adverse fetal effects.

Rubella is teratogenic with the risks being much higher in early compared with later pregnancy. Infection in the first 4 weeks of pregnancy will lead to clinical infection in 50% of cases; in the next 2 weeks this figures falls to 25% and to 10% in the next 4 weeks. After 12 weeks the risk is <1%.

Anomalies occur affecting mainly the ears, eyes, and heart. These include, in decreasing frequency; sensorineural deafness; cataracts, retinopathy and microphthalmia; central nervous system (CNS) defects; and cardiac defects (patent ductus arteriosus, pulmonary stenosis). Mental retardation is also a significant risk.

Key Practice Points

- All women should be screened for rubella immunity at booking.
- Those who are non immune should be given postnatal immunisation and advised to avoid possible contacts.
- Any pregnant women with a non vesicular rash should be investigated for rubella and parvovirus.

Hepatitis B

Routine universal antenatal screening for hepatitis B virus is currently recommended.[7] Hepatitis B virus is blood borne and very infectious. It is spread by contact with bodily secretions, e.g. through sexual intercourse, blood transfusion, intravenous drug abuse (IVDA) and perinatally. When identified, contact tracing and testing for other STIs should be initiated unless infection was known to be acquired in infancy. This should include tests for hepatitis C and HIV. It is prevalent in immigrant populations with rates as high as 1:100 in some inner city areas.

Maternal

The infection may be asymptomatic. If symptoms are present they include general symptoms (fatigue, headache and malaise) and gastrointestinal symptoms (nausea, vomiting, diarrhoea, pain in the right upper quadrant over the liver).

Signs include enlarged liver and spleen and lymphadenopathy.

Investigations may reveal raised white cell count with anaemia and thrombocytopenia. Liver function tests will show raised transaminases. Serology provides diagnostic and prognostic information. There are three structural antigens: HbsAg (surface), HbcAg (core) and HbeAg. The diagnosis of the acute infection is made by detection of hepatitis B surface antigen (HbsAg) and IgM antibody to core antigen (HbcAg) from maternal blood samples. The presence of 'e' antigens (HbeAg) is evidence of active viral replication and shedding and thus high infectivity. The presence of antibodies to the 'e' antigen (antiHbE) indicates low infectivity. Resolution of the disease is evident when antibodies to the surface (s) antigen (antiHbS) are present. The patient is then immune to the disease.

Regular monitoring for liver disease is necessary. At 3 months up to 10% of cases will have persistent HbsAg and should receive follow-up by a hepatologist as serious long-term morbidity is possible.

If detected on routine booking tests, further serology is required and referral should be made to a hepatologist.

Infection will lead to fulminant hepatitis and death in <1% of infected adults. Most (85–90%) will recover fully and antibodies will protect from further infection. The remaining 10–15% develop chronic infection with a third of these developing chronic active hepatitis or cirrhosis.

There is no contraindication to invasive testing (e.g. amniocentesis), although the available data are sparse, that which is available suggests risks of infection are low. There is also no contraindication to vaginal delivery.

Fetal and neonatal

Hepatitis B is not teratogenic, nor is the course of the infection influenced by the pregnancy. Spread to the fetus is mainly at delivery, thus in the potentially infectious woman in labour the membranes should remain intact and invasive procedures should be avoided. Non-invasive monitoring should be employed and fetal scalp sampling avoided. If assisted delivery is required, the forceps are recommended. Perinatal transmission occurs in up to 20% of cases without prophylaxis of the neonate if the mother has HbsAg, but this proportion rises to 90% if HbeAg is also present. Most of these latter cases will become chronic carriers and are therefore at increased risk of developing carcinoma of the liver or cirrhosis. Postnatal immunisation can reduce the risks of transmission by 95%, thus these babies require immunoglobulin to confer passive immunisation within 24 hours of birth as well as vaccination.

If the mother is of low infectivity—having antibodies to HbsAg and antiHbE positive—or for babies going home to an at risk environment, hepatitis B vaccine alone is required.

Any case identified antenatally should be notified to the paediatric team.

Breast feeding is acceptable in the immunised baby.

Key Practice Points

- Hepatitis B is not teratogenic but is very infective with transmission rates of up to 90% at birth.

Key Practice Points—cont'd

- Hepatitis B screening is routinely offered at booking.
- If hepatitis B positive, hepatitis C and HIV screening should be offered and other STIs considered.
- There is no evidence that invasive procedures lead to transmission, but the available data are sparse.
- Pregnancy management should include a hepatologist for new or complicated presentations.
- Paediatricians should be informed antenatally and a postnatal plan for immunisation drafted.
- At-risk neonates receive appropriate postnatal immunisation/vaccination.
- Contacts should be screened and receive vaccination.
- Vaginal delivery is acceptable but fetal blood sampling and fetal scalp electrodes should be avoided in the potentially infectious woman.

Hepatitis C

The hepatitis C virus (HCV) can be transmitted by sexual contact, blood transfusion and perinatally. It is prevalent amongst intravenous drug abusers and this is the commonest form of acquisition. Up to 2% of women are affected.

The signs of infection are non specific. Transaminases may be raised. Long-term liver damage (cirrhosis) occurs in up to 40% of patients with 3:100 developing primary liver carcinoma per annum. Unlike hepatitis B, a significant number of infected individuals (four out of five) develop chronic infection. Treatment is available with alpha interferon and ribavirin which can reduce the risk of chronic infection if commenced early in the course of infection. However, this has adverse fetal effects and is therefore contraindicated in pregnancy. Because of this, if the diagnosis is suspected in a patient in a high-risk group or with mildly raised liver function tests, serology should be tested.

Maternal

HCV is not part of routine screening; however, testing in high-risk groups should be performed. This would include anyone positive for hepatitis B or HIV. Transmission to the fetus is possible, occurring in up to 5% of cases in the UK. This will be higher if co-existent HIV is present or if there is a high titre of viral RNA in maternal serum. All such patients require combined care in pregnancy by both an obstetrician and a hepatologist. Recent evidence indicates that HCV can deteriorate in pregnancy. In addition, in advanced disease, the hepatic dysfunction may lead to thrombocytopenia, coagulopathy and portal hypertension.

Similarly to hepatitis B infection there is no evidence that invasive procedures such as chorionic villus sampling, amniocentesis and fetal blood sampling increase the risk of transmission but the data are sparse.

Fetal and neonatal

The labour management is as for hepatitis B (see above). Breast feeding does not increase risks for the neonate and is thus encouraged. There is no evidence that HCV is teratogenic, or predisposes to miscarriage or premature labour.

There is no vaccine or immunisation available for the neonate.

Key Practice Points

- Women with hepatitis B, HIV or who are known drug users should be offered hepatitis C screening.
- A patient with hepatitis C should be investigated for co-existent disease.
- The finding of raised liver function tests should prompt screening for hepatitis B and C.
- Multidisciplinary management should include an obstetrician and a hepatologist.
- There is no contraindication to vaginal delivery but fetal blood sampling and fetal scalp electrodes should be avoided.
- There is no contraindication to breast feeding.

Human immunodeficiency virus (HIV)[8]

HIV is a growing problem in the developing world. Overall 2 million HIV positive women become pregnant each year. A third of the children become infected and most will not survive to their teens. In the developed world HIV has become more manageable with reduction in vertical transmission through artificial feeding, avoidance of vaginal delivery and the use of antiretroviral therapy.

HIV is transmitted through sexual intercourse, blood transfusion and by vertical transmission from mother to child. It is estimated that 98% of children with HIV acquired this at delivery or from breast feeding.

Maternal

Routine screening for HIV has been offered for the past 2 years. This is on the basis of an opt out programme. Robust procedures are required to ensure that any positive results are followed up. Counselling of an HIV positive individual should be carried out by an appropriately trained practitioner and include discussion of the importance of antiretroviral treatment, avoidance of breast feeding, and probable avoidance of vaginal delivery unless the viral load is very low. Together these interventions can reduce neonatal transmission to 1%. Further care should include input from specialist nurses and genitourinary physicians as well as the obstetrician. In particular, it is vital that an individualised treatment plan is made to include antenatal, intrapartum and postpartum care. Unfortunately there is still a stigma attached to HIV infection in some sections of society. Confidentiality must be respected, although information should be shared between health workers. As the disease may have been acquired from intravenous drug use, consideration should be given to psychiatric referral and social work referral would also be appropriate. The association of HIV with other sexually transmitted diseases is such that screening for hepatatis B and C (including liver function tests) chlamydia, gonorrhoea and BV should be carried out. Cytomegalovirus (CMV) and toxoplasmosis can reactivate in affected individuals therefore serology should be obtained. The most important measures include regular assessment of the viral load and cluster designated (CD)4 count (CD4s are a type of cymphocyte that can decrease in number in HIV) as these will indicate disease activity and guide decisions for delivery.

Antiretroviral therapy commenced prior to pregnancy should be maintained. If HIV is diagnosed in pregnancy treatment should be individualised. The long-course zidovudine regime is commenced in the second trimester (>14 weeks) and continued through to delivery, when it is given intravenously. Following delivery it is commenced in the neonate and treatment is continued for up to 6 weeks. Such treatment reduces transmission rate to around 8%. This regimen has a good safety profile for the fetus but monotherapy is prone to viral resistance. Other drug regimens, including highly active antiretroviral therapy (HAART) which involves use of combination (3 or more drugs) therapy, suggest transmission rates of 5% or less. In general, women who require treatment for their health should be managed as for non-pregnant patients and this usually involves HAART.

HAART can lead to lactic acidosis which may present in a similar way to pre-eclampsia, and pregnant women appear to be more susceptible to this complication of therapy. The drugs can also lead to glucose intolerance and frank diabetes. If there are signs of abnormal liver function, pre-eclampsia or cholestasis, drug toxicity should be considered.

For women who are having treatment to prevent vertical transmission, therapy starts between 28 and 32 weeks. This is usually stopped after birth but continued in the infant for 6 weeks.

In established HIV infection there is no evidence that pregnancy adversely affects long-term prognosis.

Fetal and neonatal

HIV is not teratogenic. Infection occurs in the first two trimesters in 2% of cases but 80% of transmission occurs in the last 4 weeks of pregnancy, during delivery or via breast feeding, unless the placental barrier is broken such as during antenatal invasive procedures. Without protective measures, vertical transmission may occur in up to a third of babies. The measures that may reduce this risk include antiretroviral therapy, avoidance of vaginal delivery (unless the viral load is low), and avoidance of breast feeding. There is some evidence that chlorhexidine lavage of the vagina and vitamin A supplementation may also reduce the risk of transmission.

For women who are HIV positive not taking HAART during pregnancy, and for women with a detectable plasma viral load, delivery by elective Caesarean section is of clear benefit in reducing the risk of mother-to-child HIV transmission. However, whether elective Caesarean section is of benefit in women taking HAART who have an undetectable plasma viral load at the time of delivery is uncertain.[8] Discussion needs to take place on an individual basis to establish a management plan for delivery.

A maternal blood sample should be taken for viral load at delivery. If the membranes have been ruptured for more than 4 hours, the benefits reduce but Caesarean section (if this is the intended mode of delivery) should still be carried out. At delivery the umbilical cord should be clamped as soon as possible and the baby bathed. The factors that increase and decrease vertical transmission are given in Box 6.3. Overall, the combination of antenatal antiviral therapy and planned delivery may reduce the vertical transmission rate to 1%.

> **Box 6.3 Factors that positively and negatively affect vertical transmission of HIV infection**
>
> **Positively**
> - Advanced HIV infection
> - Low CD4 count
> - High viral load
> - Amniocentesis (invasive procedures)
> - Artificial rupture of membranes
> - Rupture of membranes >4 hours
> - Fetal scalp electrode
> - Vitamin A deficiency
> - Low birth weight
> - Presence of ulcerative genital infection
> - Prematurity
> - Vaginal bacterial infection
>
> **Negatively**
> - Low viral load
> - Use of zidovudine
> - Nevirapine use
> - Highly active antiretroviral therapy (HAART)
> - Caesarean section
> - Treatment of STI
> - Avoidance of breast feeding

Cytomegalovirus (CMV)

CMV has the potential to cause severe fetal abnormality. It is not teratogenic. Organs develop normally but the virus then lyses the cells, thus causing loss of function and the fetal disease. CMV can cause damage from primary infection equally in each trimester. It is the commonest cause of intrauterine infection in pregnancy with primary infection occurring in 1% of pregnancies. The sequelae can be severe but this only occurs in 7% of women primarily infected in pregnancy. This is because the fetus is only infected in 40% of cases and most neonates do not develop the disease.

Maternal

Up to 60% of women in developed countries and up to 100% of women from developing countries have evidence of past infection.

Transmission occurs directly by contact, including sexual activity and blood transfusion; however, most individuals are infected as children. The virus is found in all body fluids including blood, tears, saliva, vaginal fluid, stool, urine and semen. Vertical transmission is also a risk. Maternal infection is often asymptomatic but may present with malaise, fever and lymphadenopathy. CMV has no adverse maternal sequelae unless there is immunocompromise (acquired immuno deficiency syndrome (AIDS) or patients with transplants when fatal disseminated infection may occur). Mild hepatitis, thrombocytopenia and a haemolytic anaemia may also occur.

In general, treatment is symptomatic relief only. In severe infection, antiviral therapy such as ganciclovir may be used.

The diagnosis can be usually made by culture of the virus in urine. Serology can be useful to identify past infection; however, a rise in IgM can occur in reactivation therefore it cannot be used to confirm primary (and therefore more serious) infection. Fetal infection can be diagnosed using viral culture or PCR on a sample of liquor by amniocentesis (see below).

Fetal and neonatal

CMV is the commonest congenital infection. It is the leading cause of deafness and neurodevelopmental delay in children. Ten percent of infants with congenital CMV may show signs of a rash at birth with low birth weight, jaundice and hepatosplenomegaly. The major sequelae revolve around the viral effects on the fetal brain. These can include the development of microcephaly, chorioretinitis, sensorineural deafness, ventriculomegaly, cerebral atropy and calcification in the cerebrum which can manifest prenatally as a bright lateral border to the posterior ventricle.

In general, the sequelae are worse the earlier in gestation the infection occurs. The diagnosis may be suspected from ultrasound scan. This may reveal symmetrical early onset intrauterine growth restriction (IUGR), bright (echogenic) bowel or ventriculomegaly. Late on, in the third trimester, microcephaly and cerebral calcification may be seen. The absence of abnormal findings does not, however, ensure that there will be no neurological sequelae, which can make counselling difficult.

The diagnosis may be suggested from maternal serology. The presence of IgM indicates recent infection; however, it may be present in reactivation of CMV (see below). The presence of IgG for CMV effectively excludes primary, thus more serious, CMV infection and appears within 4–6 weeks of primary infection. The precise timing of infection is difficult to ascertain and these cases should be managed in consultation with a virologist.

Amniotic fluid culture or PCR may be used to diagnose fetal infection. Although the mother may have had primary CMV (as suggested by serological testing) this will lead to fetal infection in only 40% of cases. The amniotic fluid may give false-negative results if done less than 6 weeks after maternal infection or before 21 weeks' gestation. Fetal renal function is not developed sufficiently prior to this and infection of the renal tissue is required to excrete CMV.

From 5 to 10% of infected fetuses are symptomatic at birth and are at high risk (50–90%) of serious neurodevelopmental damage (microcephaly, cerebral palsy, learning difficulties and sensorineural hearing loss).[9] Only 15% of infected neonates born without symptoms have sequelae. The viral load influences prognosis, thus a large load will be indicative of a poor prognosis. Thirty percent of those neonates who are symptomatic will die in infancy.

Affected babies may be treated with ganciclovir which can reduce the risk of deafness. Intravenous administration is required. There are potentially serious side effects—thrombocytopenia and neutropenia—and animal studies suggest carcinogenicity. Despite these concerns, ganciclovir has been shown to improve outcome thus should be considered for those babies born with symptoms. Pregnant women in high-risk professions should ideally have serological testing. If non-immune there is no vaccine currently available, but avoidance of urine and saliva from infected children will help reduce risks.

Reactivation of latent CMV or reinfection is possible. Perhaps half of all congenital CMV infections are a result of reactivation. This is unusual for most viral infections as usually infection results in lifelong immunity. A fetus affected from reactivation/reinfection may develop sequelae but these are more mild than for primary infection. In particular, the severe neurological sequelae appear to be much reduced compared with primary infection; however, the risks are difficult to quantify. In the event infection is confirmed, then discussion regarding termination of pregnancy (both first and second trimester) is appropriate in view of the very poor long term outlook for affected infants after primary infection.

Perinatal infection, acquired by the baby from genital secretions as it delivers or after delivery from breast milk, is very different with an excellent prognosis. It may be difficult to differentiate between congenital and perinatal infections once the baby is born and it not possible to make a distinction after the infant is 3 weeks old.

Key Practice Points

- In primary CMV infection adverse fetal sequelae occur in 7% of cases.
- Infection is often asymptomatic and therefore may go unnoticed.
- There is no treatment (other than termination) but attempts at developing a vaccine continue.

Herpes simplex 1 and 2

Around 2% of women acquire the herpes simplex virus (HSV) during pregnancy. The subtype HSV 1 refers to the orofacial lesions and HSV type 2 to the genital infection; however, the subtypes can manifest in both areas. Up to 90% of adults have been previously exposed and have IgG antibodies to HSV 1 and/or 2. These antibodies offer a degree of protection to either subtype.

HSV requires close contact for infection to occur. The virus establishes latency in the sensory neurons and reactivation can occur at varying frequencies. The triggers for this include trauma, stress, ultraviolet light, a febrile illness and menstruation. In those who are immunocompromised, severe systemic infection may result.

Maternal

HSV is often asymptomatic in the primary attack. If skin lesions occur they usually affect the lips, eyes and face. Lesions are initially erythematous, becoming vesicular, finally ulcerating and crusting over. These may last 2 weeks and are painful. The genital infection affects the cervix and vulva in 90% of cases. There can be systemic symptoms with fever, malaise, headaches and myalgia in a third of cases. Recurrences are not as severe and there is often a prodromal phase with tingling in the affected area prior to visible lesions occurring.

The diagnosis is mainly a clinical one but swabs and culture to isolate the virus may be performed.

Treatment aims to limit the duration of outbreaks with topical or systemic acyclovir and has not been shown to be teratogenic. Analgesia and warm saline baths may help as can topical local anaesthetic gel. Rarely symptoms can be so severe that urinary retention occurs, requiring catheterisation. Hospital admission may be necessary to provide adequate analgesia.

Infection in pregnancy should be managed with advice from a genitourinary physician. Intravenous therapy may be required in primary herpes simplex infection due to the relatively immunocompromised state that pregnancy can confer. Disseminated disease with neurological, cutaneous and liver involvement is uncommon but more likely in pregnancy. This is most likely in the last two trimesters and mortality can be significant.

Antenatal management depends on the timing of infection and whether it is primary or secondary. If infection occurs in the first two trimesters there is no evidence of teratogenicity and no requirement for Caesarean section (see below).

If a primary attack develops earlier in pregnancy, treatment with suppressive doses of acyclovir (400 mg twice daily) from 36 weeks' gestation may reduce recurrence and anxiety about whether delivery by Caesarean section is necessary.

If the primary attack is within 6 weeks of delivery, intravenous acyclovir intrapartum may reduce neonatal herpes and Caesarean section should be considered, although the evidence suggests the major risk for the neonate is from infection immediately around the time of delivery, thus vaginal delivery can be considered.[10]

If a primary attack occurs at the time of delivery, Caesarean section is recommended if within 4 hours of rupture of membranes.

For recurrent infection if active lesion(s) are identified in labour the risks to the baby of neonatal herpes are small and should be set against the risks to the mother of Caesarean section.[10] It is worth noting that in the Netherlands no Caesarean section as been carried out for recurrent herpes simplex since 1987 and no adverse neonatal sequelae have been reported.[11]

For frequently recurring HSV, acyclovir from 36 weeks will reduce the risk of recurrence in labour, but this is not yet routinely recommended as there is still insufficient evidence of benefit.[10]

After delivery, direct contact between any active lesions and the baby should be avoided, but separation is not necessary.

Staff with lesions should contact their local occupational health department as advice differs, but it may be recommended that an individual remain off work until the lesions are no longer considered infective.

Fetal and neonatal

Neonatal herpes is rare, occurring in 7:100 000 live births. It is acquired from contact during vaginal delivery and is most likely when primary infection occurs near or at delivery. Perinatal transmission occurs in 40% of cases at this time. Neonatal herpes is a serious infection which can lead to high morbidity and mortality. The infection can affect the skin, eyes or mouth and lead to encephalitis and disseminated infection. Death is unusual with treatment of local infection but is commoner in systemic disease.

Key Practice Points

- Primary HSV infection can lead to serious sequelae for the fetus.
- HSV diagnosed in pregnancy should be managed with advice from a genitourinary physician.
- Infection in the first and second trimesters and secondary infections are not a contraindication to vaginal delivery.
- Primary infection at the time of delivery is an indication for Caesarean section to prevent neonatal herpes, which has serious sequelae.
- Caesarean section should take place within 4 hours of rupture of membranes.

Varicella-zoster virus (VZV, chicken pox)

Chicken pox is commonly acquired in childhood. The virus is spread by direct contact with the vesicles, via droplet spread from the upper respiratory tract. After the primary infection the virus remains latent in dorsal root ganglia. Reactivation leads to shingles which tends to occur in a dermatomal pattern. This can be infective by direct contact with vesicles.

Antenatally, history of varicella contact should be sought; most will be immune but those negative for VZV should be advised about risks and avoiding contact with infected individuals.

Maternal

Due to the high level of acquired immunity (90%) the risk of infection in pregnancy is only 0.3%.

Contact sufficient to cause infection can occur when a susceptible individual has been face-to-face for 5 minutes, in the same room (e.g. 4-bedded hospital bay) for 15 minutes, or household contact has occurred.

Unlike CMV infection there are usually symptoms with VZV infection.

There is likely to be a history of contact with an affected individual. Non-specific malaise and fever is followed by a pruritic rash on the face and trunk which is initially maculopapular, becoming vesicular with characteristic rupture of the vesicles and crusting over. The individual is infective from 2 days prior to the rash until the last vesicle crusts over, or 6 days after the rash appears, whichever is the later.

Herpes zoster, which is a reactivation, results in painful vesicles over the distribution of one sensory or motor nerve root. Systemic infection can result but this is most likely in an immunocompromised individual.

The diagnosis is a clinical one with confirmation available through serological testing, measuring IgM (for primary infection) or IgG (for past infection). Infection in childhood usually confers lifelong protection.

Vaccination is available and the effects of infection may be influenced by the use of acyclovir. Intravenous therapy will be required in systemic disease (see below). In a non-immune individual contact should prompt serological testing if not previously performed. These results can be available in 24–48 hours provided they are marked urgent. Many laboratories keep the rubella sample from booking and this can be used to test for immunity following a telephone call to the laboratory. This is useful as 90% of women who are unsure about previous infection will be found to have antibodies demonstrating immunity. If antibodies are present within 10 days of the contact, they probably pre-existed the contact. If negative and within 10 days of contact, varicella-zoster immunoglobulin (VZIG) should be administered. (This may only be available to those less than 12 weeks and over 36 weeks' gestation due to a shortage of vaccine.) This is of no benefit if varicella has developed, but reduces the severity of the disease in adults and neonates and also the risk of fetal varicella syndrome if given prior to clinical VZV infection. Up to 85% of cases will be afforded complete or at least partial protection.[12]

If the rash is less than 24 hours old then oral acyclovir (800 mg five times a day for 7 days) should be given. There is no evidence the drug is teratogenic.

If VZV develops in late pregnancy after 36 weeks, the delivery should be delayed if possible to allow the clinical course of the disease to complete, which will allow passive immunity for the neonate from maternal IgG. In the acute viraemic phase the mother is at risk of disseminated intravascular coagulation; this is another reason why delivery should be delayed until after the vesicles have finished crusting over. If presenting after 24 hours, no treatment is beneficial thus close observation for serious sequelae should be maintained.

Serious maternal complications may include encephalitis, hepatitis, continued vesicular cropping after 6 days, a dense rash and relapsing pyrexia and pneumonia. If any complication is suspected, the woman should be referred for hospital assessment. Intravenous acyclovir may be required in the immunocompromised woman or in those with complications related to VZV infection.

Pneumonia is reported in 10% of adult cases. It is most likely in smokers, in those with a chronic respiratory illness, and where prolonged steroid therapy has been used within 3 months of the VZV infection.

All women, however, should be warned to report any chest symptoms (dry or productive cough or shortness of breath either on exertion or at rest) as VZV pneumonia is a severe disease, requiring intensive care in many cases. It is a cause of maternal death in 2% of women who develop pneumonia, but in up to 40% of those requiring mechanical ventilation.

Shingles is not usually a cause for concern for the mother or baby if it is present at the time of delivery. However, in the presence of severe symptoms such as pain or in the immunocompromised woman, oral acyclovir may be appropriate. Ophthalmic zoster should also be considered for topical and systemic treatment.

Fetal and neonatal

Congenital VZV infection can lead to serious sequelae (Box 6.4). It is not the VZV itself that causes the structural effects but reactivation, resulting in a fetal herpes zoster infection that has its effects in a dermatomal distribution. As with most other viral infections, the timing of infection has a relationship to the long-term effects of the congenital infection. Infection in the first trimester (up to 12 weeks) carries a smaller risk of congenital infection of up to 0.6%. Between 13 and 20 weeks the risk is low with 1–2% of fetuses infected developing the varicella syndrome. Between 20 and 36 weeks there are few if any fetal effects; certainly the varicella syndrome does not occur.

Transplacental passage of the VZV increases with gestation, thus neonatal infection occurs in 60% of cases if maternal infection happens within 4 weeks of delivery. Infection after 36 weeks can result in the birth of a child without the benefit of maternal antibodies against VZV and severe neonatal varicella may result with serious mortality and morbidity. If the onset of maternal VZV infection is within 5 days of delivery or 2 days after delivery, the neonate is vulnerable to severe disease with a mortality of up to 30%. This risk can be attenuated by the use of a high dose varicella-zoster immunoglobulin given to the susceptible neonate. It is recommended that this should be administered to newborns where the mother has developed varicella within 7 days of delivery. A neonate developing VZV should be treated with acyclovir.

If there is evidence of infection within the first half of pregnancy, referral to a fetal medicine unit should be made due to the previously discussed risks of fetal varicella syndrome. The diagnosis can be made prenatally using ultrasound. However, anomalies do not become evident until 5 weeks or more after fetal infection. Findings may include calcification in the fetal liver and intraabdominally, ventriculomegaly, microcephaly (usually a late finding), evidence of limb malformation, symmetrical growth restriction and polyhydramnios.

Invasive procedures have limited use in confirming the diagnosis. Amniocentesis or fetal blood sampling may reveal evidence of VZV but are not diagnostic of fetal infection.

Babies of mothers who developed VZV during pregnancy but avoided the serious sequelae are at risk of herpes zoster infection in early life, but this is not usually problematic.

If a mother has developed VZV in the first 20 weeks of pregnancy, the neonate should be referred for ophthalmic assessment.

Box 6.4 Sequelae of congenital varicella syndrome with fetal infection < 20 weeks' gestation

- **Skin**
  - Cicatrisation (scarring)—dermatomal pattern
- **Eye**
  - Microphthalmia
  - Chorioretinitis
  - Cataracts
- **Limbs**
  - Hypoplasia
- **Neurological**
  - Microcephaly
  - Cortical atrophy
  - Mental retardation
  - Bowel and bladder sphincter dysfunction

Key Practice Points

- A history of previous chicken pox infection should be taken at booking.
- Those with no previous history should be advised to avoid contacts and seek medical advice if contact occurs.
- If contact occurs in pregnancy, prior immunity can often be checked on a booking sample or urgent serology can be sent.
- If VZV infection has been acquired in pregnancy, the patient should avoid contact with susceptible individuals and also avoid the maternity unit.
- Any visitors to infective women should be immune and this includes medical and midwifery staff.
- If a child at home has VZV the immune mother will have conferred passive immunity to her newborn and thus there is little risk.
- If a child at home has VZV and the mother is not immune, the neonate should receive VZIG, the mother acyclovir.

Key Practice Points—cont'd

- Chicken pox infection in pregnancy can lead to serious maternal morbidity and mortality and medical advice should be sought, particularly if there are respiratory symptoms.
- Fetal infection between 13 and 20 weeks carries 1–2% risk of varicella syndrome; infection in the latter weeks of pregnancy may lead to neonatal varicella.
- Maternal infection 5 days before or 2 days after delivery risks neonatal infection.
- Neonates should receive VZIG if delivered within 7 days of maternal infection.
- Infected neonates should receive acyclovir.

Human parvovirus B19 (HPVB19)[13]

Alternatively known as fifth disease, slapped cheek and erythema infectiosum, this is a benign disease in children and adults. It mostly affects infant school children with outbreaks occurring every 3 years. Its significance is its effect when acquired in pregnancy. Although not teratogenic, it can have profound effects on the fetus leading to mortality if unrecognised.

Maternal

The virus is spread by respiratory droplets. Up to 50% of adults show evidence of past infection. Susceptible individuals have a 50% chance of infection after household exposure and 30% after exposure at school/nursery. Infection in children is mild with general malaise, fever and the characteristic facial rash, the slapped cheek. Adults may also have a rash (face, trunk and limbs) but also can develop arthralgia. By the time the rash appears, the subject is no longer infective. There are no serious sequelae except in the immunocompromised or patients with high red cell turnover, e.g. sickle cell disease. The diagnosis is by serology.

If maternal infection is suspected or confirmed, serial weekly ultrasound should be commenced looking for signs of hydrops fetalis or for signs of fetal anaemia using Doppler assessment of the fetal middle cerebral artery. Surveillance should be continued for 12 weeks for women with serologically confirmed infection.

Fetal and neonatal

Infection in the first 20 weeks of gestation can lead to spontaneous miscarriage and intrauterine death (without hydrops fetalis). The diagnosis of HPVB19 in pregnancy requires referral to a fetal medicine unit for appropriate care. If acquired in pregnancy, there is a 25% chance of transplacental spread. There is a 3–9% fetal loss rate after infection. The risks appear highest when infection is acquired between 12 and 20 weeks. The virus has a predilection for the erythroid progenitor cells in the fetal bone marrow, causing anaemia, but pancytopenia may also occur. This is effected through the P antigen to which the virus binds. These are present on the myocardium, thus in a quarter of cases a myocarditis develops also. The fetus develops hydrops fetalis from high output failure secondary to fetal anaemia with cardiac dysfunction exacerbating the condition. This can develop up to 18 weeks after the original infection but usually develops within 3–8 weeks.

The diagnosis is made from maternal serology. If negative for IgM and IgG but there is a good history of exposure, a sample should be retaken 3–4 weeks later for evidence of seroconversion.

Diagnosis also can be made by fetal serology on blood sampling (but IgM is only detectable after 22 weeks) and PCR (also possible with an amniocentesis sample) to detect evidence of viral infection.

Treatment of the fetus is with in utero transfusion to correct fetal anaemia, allowing a good outcome in most cases (>85%). Spontaneous recovery can occur and most fetuses do not have long-term sequelae as a result.

Key Practice Points

- Pregnant women developing a non-vesicular rash in pregnancy should be investigated for HPVB19 (and rubella) irrespective of previous tests.
- Contact face-to-face or same room for 15 minutes with non-vesicular rash (or prior to that person developing the rash) should also prompt testing.
- Referral to a fetal medicine centre should be made following a diagnosis of HPVB19 in pregnancy.
- Human parvovirus B19 is not teratogenic but has its fetal effects by causing fetal anaemia and/or a myocarditis which may lead to fetal loss with or without hydrops fetalis.

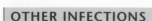

OTHER INFECTIONS

Toxoplasmosis

The incidence of toxoplasmosis acquired in pregnancy is between 1 and 2:1000. The definitive host for this intracellular parasite is the cat. Spread most commonly occurs via ingestion of raw/undercooked meat (e.g. pigs (including Parma/Serrano ham) or sheep that have ingested contaminated food) or from soil or cat litter contaminated with faeces. Up to 85% of women are susceptible to infection in the UK.

Maternal

The infection is often asymptomatic. Any symptoms will be non-specific with fever, malaise, tiredness and lymphadenopathy. There are no significant long-term sequelae except in the immunocompromised and those with HIV infection. These latter may experience chorioretinitis, pneumonitis, encephalitis and reactivation of latent infection in the central nervous system.

In addition the fetus is at risk of congenital infection.

Detection is by serological testing, and infected individuals may be offered treatment in pregnancy with spiramycin (see below).

Advice should be given on how to avoid infection as routine testing is not carried out in the UK.[3] Risk of disease comes from contact with cat faeces. Therefore pregnant women should wear gloves for gardening and avoid dealing with cat litter if possible. Meat should be handled with care and well cooked. If infection is suspected then serology can be performed, but interpretation can be problematic as the IgM can stay present for up to 2 years. Confirmatory testing is carried out at a toxoplasma reference laboratory in cases shown positive for toxoplasma infection. Invasive testing can be useful with PCR on amniotic fluid proving a reliable test. Ultrasound can be used to diagnose serious sequelae, but a normal scan will not ensure normal outcome; indeed, 90% of cases will be subclinical at birth and thus undetectable by ultrasound.

In suspected cases spiramycin should be commenced whilst awaiting confirmatory tests. If confirmed then spiramycin is alternated with sulfadiazine and pyrimethamine. The extent to which this helps is unclear but it does reduce serious sequelae (see below).

Termination may be offered if the infection occurred at a time of high risk for congenital infection or there is evidence of severe disease on ultrasound.

Fetal and neonatal

Infection in the first trimester occurs in 6–25% of cases and transmisson rates rise throughout gestation until the late third trimester when it may occur in up to 90%. However, first trimester infection leads to serious sequelae—the classic triad of chorioretinitis, hydrocephalus and intracranial calcification—in 60% of cases compared with 9% at 36 weeks. Other manifestations include intrauterine growth restriction and hepatosplenomegaly.

> ### Key Practice Points
>
> - Pregnant women should be advised to avoid raw/undercooked meat including Parma/Serrano ham.
> - Pregnant women should be advised to wear gloves when gardening and avoid dealing with cat litter.
> - Routine testing is not performed in the UK and serology interpretation can be difficult (IgM stays positive for up to 2 years).
> - Invasive testing may be required to obtain a diagnosis.
> - Treatment can alleviate but not prevent sequelae.

Chlamydia

This is now the commonest STI. It is prevalent among the young, those with multiple partners and in those in a low socioeconomic group and with other STIs. There are often no symptoms (75%) but infection can lead to devastating sequelae, commonly subfertility, which may occur in 1 in 10 women after one episode of chlamydia related pelvic inflammatory disease. There is also a strong association with ectopic pregnancy. Currently any screening is opportunistic at genitourinary clinics or in those women seeking termination of pregnancy. In the near future any woman under the age of 25 presenting to antenatal clinic will be offered screening.[3]

Maternal

If symptoms are present they may include vaginal discharge, intermenstrual/abnormal vaginal bleeding, dyspareunia, abdominal pain and dysuria. Some of these are unreliable in the pregnant patient. The main maternal complication seen with chlamydial infection is postpartum endometritis.

Where infection is suspected or in an at-risk individual, an endocervical swab or first void urine are suitable samples for testing. If testing is positive, care should be continued by a genitourinary clinic that can arrange appropriate contact tracing and patient follow-up. Treatment in pregnancy should be with erythromycin 500 mg 6-hourly for 7 days (as tetracyclines are contraindicated). Amoxycillin 500 mg 8-hourly for 7 days is a suitable alternative. Otherwise azithromycin (which has the advantage of being a once only dose), or clindamycin are alternatives.

A test of cure should always be performed as erythromycin and amoxicillin will only result in a cure in 85% of cases.

Fetal and neonatal

Chlamydial infections are probably associated with premature labour, PPROM and low birth weight but the evidence is conflicting. In an untreated mother the neonate can develop conjunctivitis (50%). This occurs late (6–12 days) compared with the opthalmia neonatorum from gonococcal infection, which occurs at day 2. A pneumonitis may occur in up to 20% of cases. This usually manifests 3–12 weeks postnatally as respiratory compromise.

Key Practice Points

- Currently screening for chlamydia in pregnancy is not recommended but this may change.
- The Chlamydia Advisory Group recommended that women under 25, or over 25 with a new sexual partner or who have had two partners in 12 months should be offered screening.
- Confirmed cases should be referred for genitourinary follow-up.
- Post treatment testing should also be performed as cure rates are lower in pregnancy.
- It is a prevalent condition with significant neonatal and maternal sequelae that can be easily treated.

Syphilis[3]

Syphilis is caused by a spirochaete *Treponema pallidum* through sexual intercourse. It had become much less common with few cases identified per annum, however, nationally the incidence is now increasing. Screening for the disease is still part of routine antenatal care. Untreated, it can progress to serious long-term morbidity.

Maternal

After initial infection the disease spreads rapidly. The chancre is the initial lesion. It is a raised, small painless ulcer (primary syphilis) and this stage can be missed through lack of symptoms. Untreated, this progresses to secondary syphilis in most patients and this results in systemic effects with pyrexia, general malaise, a rash, mucosal lesions and lymphadenopathy. This can occur 3 weeks to 3 months after primary infection. Further progression to tertiary syphilis occurs in a third of untreated cases after a latent period of variable timing—several years can pass between secondary and tertiary stages. Tertiary syphilis can affect the nervous system, the heart or lead to gummatous disease.

Serology is the diagnostic method of choice as the spirochaete is not easy to culture. These tests are of two types, non-treponemal and treponemal. The initial venereal disease research laboratory (VDRL) and the raid plasma reagin (RPR) are sensitive thus

Box 6.5 Causes of false-positive results from VDRL and RPR tests for syphilis

- **Acute viral illness**
  - Hepatitis
  - Measles
- **Infections**
  - Tuberculosis
  - Other spirochaetes (e.g. Yaws)
  - Malaria
- **Malignancy**
- **Pregnancy**
- **Autoimmune disease**
  - Systemic lupus erythematosis

useful for screening. If positive, confirmatory tests that are specific such as the fluorescent-treponemal antibody-absorbed test (FTA-ABS) allow accurate diagnosis. It is important to realise that false-positives may occur with the screening tests offered in routine antenatal care (Box 6.5). After confirmation of a reactive specimen, a second sample should be tested to verify results.

The treatment depends on the length of infection. If present for less than 1 year, one intramuscular injection of penicillin is curative, with larger doses if infected for longer. The treatment should be conducted by a specialist in genitourinary medicine to ensure contact tracing is performed.

Fetal and neonatal

The risk of fetal infection is greatest in the initial stages of the disease as the spirochetaemia is at its greatest. Syphilis can be acquired transplacentally throughout pregnancy from 9 weeks or by direct contact with a genital lesion. Untreated, its effects are severe leading to miscarriage and an increased perinatal mortality rate of 60% with half stillborn and half dying in the neonatal period. The remainder develop late syphilis. It can lead to preterm labour and is a cause of non-immune hydrops fetalis and IUGR.

Infection by congenital syphilis may be regarded as early (less than 2 years) and late, often occurring around puberty.

Infection in pregnancy may be investigated by invasive testing. PCR of liquor is very sensitive and specific. Fetal blood may be used also, and can

identify IgM to *T. pallidum* which must therefore be fetally produced. Ultrasound will identify hydrops fetalis, bowel dilatation, an enlarged placenta and hepatosplenomegaly, which is the single most consistent sign. The condition is identifiable from 20 weeks.

Even if appropriately treated, 15% of infected fetuses will die or be delivered with congenital syphilis.[14]

Key Practice Points

- Syphilis screening is part of routine antenatal care.
- Evidence of infection should prompt referral to genitourinary medicine.
- Untreated syphilis has serious maternal, fetal and neonatal consequences.
- Syphilis cases are rising in all groups of society.

Listeria

Listeria monocytogenes is carried in 10% of humans in the gut. This will rarely cause problems in the healthy individual; however, in the immunocompromised (including HIV), fetus/newborn and pregnant woman illness may be severe.

Maternal

Infection comes from various foodstuffs and part of the antenatal care received should include advice on avoidance of unpasteurised milk, rinded soft cheese, pâté, and to wash pre-bagged salads and vegetables. Advice on simple measures such as washing vegetables well to reduce the risk of infection should be given. Reheated rice and ready made meals are also associated with *Listeria monocytogenes* infection. Ready meals must be thoroughly heated before consumption.

An infected individual may have no symptoms or a flu-like illness with pyrexia, and gastrointestinal symptoms such as nausea and vomiting. In advanced disease the patient may develop septicaemia or an encephalitis.

The diagnosis can be made from blood cultures and stool samples. Serological testing may be helpful.

The antibiotic of choice is penicillin.

Fetal and neonatal

Listeria monocytogenes is associated with miscarriage, premature labour and stillbirth. A peculiarity of *L. monocytogenes* infection is the presence of meconium stained liquor at early gestation in affected cases. Thus if present at gestations less than 34 weeks, listeriosis should be suspected.

A congenitally infected neonate can be very ill with pneumonia, hepatomegaly and meningitis present at birth or developing within 24 hours of delivery. A typical finding is of pink/grey granulomas on the skin. Neonatal mortality may reach 15%. Treatment of infection is with ampicillin and gentamycin.

Key Practice Points

- All pregnant women should be advised to avoid unpasteurised milk, soft cheese, raw meat and pre-bagged salads and vegetables.

CONCLUSION

This is not a comprehensive review of all the infections that can affect pregnancy but the most important have been included. The detection of certain infections is already part of routine antenatal screening with more likely to be introduced in the near future (e.g. chlamydia).

In many cases the maternal infection may go unrecognised and there are often no adverse sequelae for the mother (an obvious exception being VZV pneumonia). This may mean that the supposed frequency of adverse fetal sequelae is in fact much lower than currently estimated as many transplacental infections go unrecognised. Unfortunately the developing fetus may not fare as well. In general, infection in the first trimester leads to more severe sequelae (which may include neurodevelopmental delay, microcephaly, hydrocephalus, blindness and deafness) compared with infection in the second and third trimesters.

If infection is suspected then serology should be undertaken with the presence of IgM suggesting recent infection, and IgG past infection and immunity. In many cases patients will be immune to the infection (e.g. VZV infection) and can be reassured as reinfection is uncommon and usually less severe in its effects. If serology is negative then further investigation is required, thus referral to a centre specialising in fetal medicine is important. Invasive procedures may be offered to aid diagnosis, with frequent ultrasound scans looking for evidence of fetal infection.

Some infections are amenable to treatment which may not cure but may limit the effects of disease.

A particular group that are susceptible are the immunocompromised, including those with HIV. As more women with organ transplants are achieving pregnancy and treatments for HIV improve survival and reduce risks to the unborn child, this group is likely to attain more significance. This may see an increase in prenatal infection rate. In the future vaccines for some of the infections discussed will become available. More will become the subject of screening, with more rapid reliable screening and diagnostic tests also being developed. It is hoped this will lead to a reduction in the number of babies born with severe congenital infection.

References

1. Royal College of Obstetricians and Gynaecologists. Prevention of early onset neonatal group B streptococcal disease. Guideline No. 36. London: RCOG; 2003.
2. Smaill F. Intrapartum antibiotics for group B streptococcal colonisation. Cochrane Database Syst Rev 2000; CD000115.
3. National Collaborating Centre for Women's and Children's Health. Antenatal care: routine care for the healthy pregnant woman. Clinical Guideline No. 6. London: RCOG; 2003.
4. Romero R, Oyarzun E, Mazor M, et al. Meta-analysis of the relationship between asymptomatic bacteriuria and preterm delivery/low birth weight. Obstet Gynecol 1989; 73:576–582.
5. Hay PE, Lamont RF, Taylor-Robinson D, et al. Abnormal bacterial colonisation of the genital

tract as a marker for subsequent preterm delivery and late miscarriage. BMJ 1994; 308:295–298.

6. Murphy DJ, Sellers S, Mackenzie IZ, et al. Case-control study of antenatal and intrapartum risk factors for cerebral palsy in very preterm singleton babies. Lancet 1995; 346:1449–1454.

7. UK National Screening Committee. Screening of pregnant women for hepatitis B and immunisation of babies at risk. Health Services Circular 1998/127. London: Department of Health; 1998.

8. Royal College of Obstetricians and Gynaecologists. Management of HIV in pregnancy. Guideline No.39. London: RCOG; 2004.

9. Ramsey MEB, Miller E, Peckham CS. Outcome of confirmed symptomatic congential CMV infection. Arch Dis Child 1991; 66:1068–1069.

10. Royal College of Obstetricians and Gynaecologists. Management of genital herpes in pregnancy. Guideline No.30. London: RCOG; 2002.

11. Van Everdinger JJ, Peeters MF, ten Have P. Neonatal herpes policy in The Netherlands. Five years after a consensus conference. J Perinat Med 1993; 21:371–375.

12. Royal College of Obstetricians and Gynaecologists. Chicken pox in pregnancy. Guideline No.13. London: RCOG; 2001.

13. Von Kaisenberg CS. Jonat W. Fetal parvovirus B19 infection. Ultrasound Obstet Gynecol 2001; 18:280–288.

14. Conover CS, Rend CA, Miller GB Jr, Schmid GP. Congenital syphilis after treatment of maternal syphilis with a penicillin regimen exceeding CDC guidelines. Infect Dis Obstet Gynecol 1998; 6:134–137.

Section Three

Fetal investigations

SECTION CONTENTS

7

First trimester ultrasound scans

Ann Minton, Donna Holdcroft

INTRODUCTION

As ultrasound technology has developed, practitioners have been able to identify both major structural abnormalities, such as spina bifida,[1] and also more subtle indicators known as 'markers'. Markers can be indicative of an underlying congenital abnormality.[2]

The ability to view the fetus from an early age coupled with issues of obstetric welfare have led to an increasing wish by parents and clinicians to identify potential anomalies earlier than the 20 week anomaly scan, which is offered to most women antenatally. Thus, pregnancy can now be assessed in the first trimester not only for viability, gestational number and age (i.e. quantitative assessment), but qualitative assessments about fetal structure and abnormality can now also be made, with some degree of accuracy.[3,4] Figure 7.1 summarises how ultrasound is used in the first trimester to manage pregnancy problems and is useful to refer to throughout the chapter.

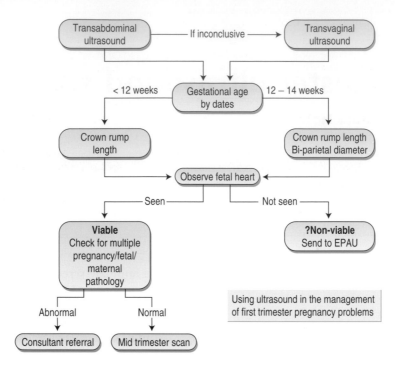

Figure 7.1 Using ultrasound in the management of first trimester pregnancy problems.

Dating scans

The purpose of the dating scan is to assess viability, assess the number of fetuses, identify any maternal or fetal pathology if present and to determine an accurate gestational age of the fetus.

Dates by scan and last menstrual period

Traditionally the expected date of confinement was calculated from the first day of the last menstrual period, with days being added or subtracted for long or short cycles. There is now ample evidence from ultrasound studies achieved with assisted conception techniques (i.e. where the exact length of pregnancy at the time of scan is known) that the commonly used ultrasound formulae are accurate.[5] There is good epidemiological evidence that ultrasound dates alone better predict the expected date of delivery than 'certain' menstrual dates alone or in combination with scan dates.[6] Dating error is important overall, but especially at the extremes of pregnancy.[7] National Institute of Clinical Excellence

(NICE) guidelines suggest that dating scans are performed between 10 and 13 weeks and use crown–rump length measurement to determine gestational age. Scan measurements should always be used when performing serum screening for Down's syndrome.

In early pregnancy misdating can result in an error in counselling and, at the other extreme, post-dated pregnancies may result in unnecessary labour inductions. Preference of scan dates over menstrual dates does not signify questioning of the first day of the mother's last menstrual period but merely an uncertainty about the day of conception. It is note-worthy that the date of conception may differ from the date of ovulation and sexual intercourse. Mothers should be counselled appropriately. From the evidence it is recommended that pregnancies are dated in the first trimester by ultrasound alone.

Measurements

Dating by ultrasound in the first trimester can be undertaken by measuring either the gestation sac volume (GSV), crown–rump Length (CRL) or biparietal diameter (BPD). Gestation can be calculated using GSV but the method is inaccurate and there is a lack of dating charts available. For this reason the CRL and BPD are preferred.

The embryo can be visualised from about 6 weeks' gestation by transabdominal scanning and cardiac activity can normally be detected by the time the embryo can be resolved by the ultrasound machine. Correctly performed CRL measurements are the most accurate means of assessing gestational age (see Fig. 7.2).

The evidence of accuracy of first trimester dating by crown–rump length extends only to about 11 weeks as the fetus sometimes becomes flexed and so a true longitudinal section is difficult to obtain. The accuracy of the CRL depends upon the operator's ability to obtain a true longitudinal section of the fetus with both the end points clearly visible. Errors can be made in the measurement if the fetus is flexed or the yolk sac is inadvertently included in the measurement. The dates by ultrasound scan performed between 6 and 11 weeks should be accurate to within 5 days.

The BPD can be measured from approximately 12 weeks' gestation and should always be measured at the correct level and section outlined in the British Medical Ultrasound (BMUS) chart, that includes a short midline in the anterior two thirds of the head, the cavum septum pellucidum and the basal cisterns (see Fig. 7.3). Sometimes the fetus will lie with its head down in the maternal pelvis, making an appropriate section difficult to obtain. If this is the case then the woman's bladder must be filled or a transvaginal scan performed to obtain the correct section. Major head abnormalities are associated with chromosome abnormalities and detecting them at an early gestation maximises the options open to the woman, so an appropriate section to obtain a BPD measurement is preferable to a CRL measurement. Evidence on accuracy of BPD is from 14–15 weeks only.

There are currently no studies that have looked at the error of biometry dating at 12–14 weeks.[8] Therefore, until evidence emerges, dates derived from a scan during this interval are best reviewed again with the result of the 18–20 week scan. After approximately 14–15 weeks, BPD in conjunction with femur length (FL) should be used to assess gestational age. However, NICE guidelines suggest that for women scanned before 24 weeks, irrespective of measurement method, using dating by ultrasound is sufficiently accurate to reduce the number of births to be considered post-term.

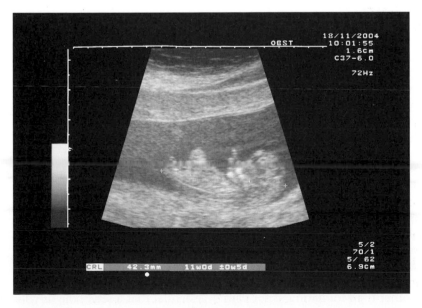

Figure 7.2 Crown–rump length measurement 11 weeks.

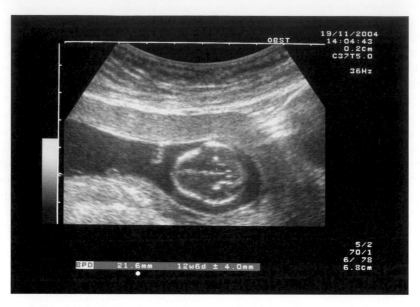

Figure 7.3   Biparietal diameter (BPR) measurement at 12 weeks 6 days.

Prediction of gestational age by ultrasound is not accurate after 24 weeks' gestation. In women presenting after 24 weeks' gestation a growth scan should be performed at a 2-week interval to determine fetal growth. It should be possible to give an estimated date of confinement after the second scan. It must be recognised that this is an estimate and decisions regarding intervention must encompass the clinical context.

Viability

Unfortunately not all ultrasound scans for dating go to plan. Women may present for dating with bleeding or pain, or sometimes mothers may be asymptomatic. Much research has been carried out regarding the accuracy of ultrasound in assessing fetal viability and guidelines have been established[9] to assist staff with decision making when scan reports for viability are equivocal. These guidelines were written as a result of a potential tragedy involving the inaccurate reporting of fetal loss. Fortunately, the ultrasound scan was repeated and the woman did not undergo an evacuation of products of conception.[9]

The most common reason for referral for scan in the first trimester, other than for dating, is for pain or bleeding. A full pelvic survey should be undertaken initially, with a full bladder, on every woman. If enough detail cannot be seen then it is usual to proceed to a transvaginal scan with the woman's consent. Even in early pregnancy when the operator feels sure that a transvaginal scan will be needed, it is still better to start with a transabdominal approach as some appearances of ectopic pregnancy and ovarian cysts may not be as clear on transvaginal scan.

Details recorded on the ultrasound report should include the number of sacs and the mean gestation age sac diameter, the regularity of the sac outline, the presence of haematoma, the presence of a yolk sac, the presence of a fetal pole, the crown–rump measurement and the presence or absence of fetal heart movements.

COMMON ULTRASOUND FINDINGS

This section describes some common early pregnancy ultrasound findings.

Ongoing intrauterine pregnancy

To be sure that the pregnancy is in the uterus it is essential that a fetal pole or yolk sac is clearly identified within the uterine cavity. If only a sac is visualised in the uterus, without any fetal contents, then caution must be exercised as sometimes an ectopic pregnancy may also have an intrauterine pseudo sac, which may be misinterpreted as an early intrauterine pregnancy. This highlights the importance of ensuring that fetal parts or yolk sac are visualised to exclude misinterpretation.

Sometimes, in women with bleeding, haemorrhage may be seen adjacent to the gestation sac which can explain the reason for the bleeding/pain. However, in most cases no cause for the symptoms are identified on the scan. It is therefore important that, when referring women for a scan for symptoms, this is clearly understood. Many women are disappointed to find that the ultrasound cannot find a cause for pain or bleeding.

Missed miscarriage

There are many appearances of a missed miscarriage on ultrasound scan.

The main two are described below:

1. Fetal pole (see Fig. 7.4) is seen without evidence of a fetal heart beat. Caution must be applied in these cases. The scan should be undertaken using a transvaginal approach. The Royal College of Radiologists (RCR) and Royal College of Obstetricians and Gynaecologists (RCOG) guideline[9] stipulates that fetal death cannot be confirmed with confidence if the CRL of the fetus is less than 6 mm. In cases where the fetal pole measures less than this, then a repeat scan should be undertaken to assess growth after 7–14 days and to establish whether heart activity exists. Women may be counselled that the ultrasound appearances are highly suggestive of missed miscarriage. Some operators may also apply colour Doppler as confirmation that there is no movement within the fetus.

2. If the gestation sac has a mean sac diameter greater than 20 mm, with no evidence of an embryo or yolk sac, this is highly suggestive of an anembryonic pregnancy (formerly known as a blighted ovum) (see Fig. 7.5). Once again, if the mean diameter of the gestation sac is smaller than this then a repeat scan to assess viability is recommended.

Ectopic pregnancy

The term ectopic pregnancy can be used to describe any pregnancy situated outside the endometrial cavity and is the cause of approximately 10% of direct maternal deaths.[10] At-risk groups include

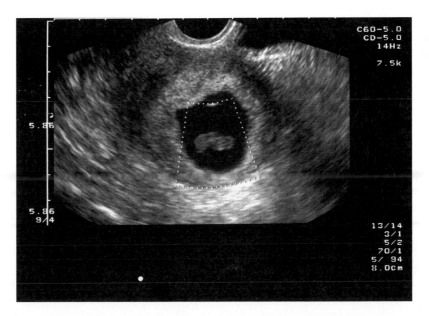

Figure 7.4 Fetal pole.

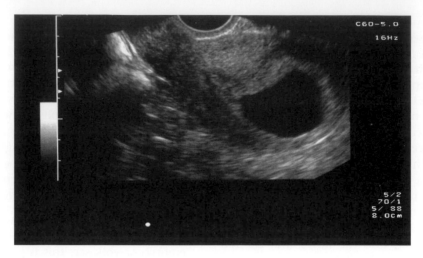

Figure 7.5 Anembryonic pregnancy.

women with pelvic inflammatory disease, adhesions or endometriosis, women who have an intrauterine contraceptive device (IUCD), and women who have undergone artificial insemination. It can also be one of the most difficult pathologies to diagnose on ultrasound examination, due to the large number of ultrasound features. Only 10% of ectopic pregnancies[11] can be seen as having a fetus outside the uterine cavity. (see Fig. 7.6). The others usually have variable appearances (e.g. mass/cyst, etc.) and a lack of pregnancy in the uterine cavity. Therefore any woman presenting with a positive pregnancy test and in which a pregnancy cannot be clearly identified within the uterine cavity must be considered as being at risk of having an ectopic pregnancy.

There are some ultrasound signs that may raise the suspicion of an ectopic pregnancy, such as free fluid being present in the pouch of Douglas or adnexal mass (between the uterus and ovaries); however, the gold standard for diagnosis remains a laparoscopy.

Complete miscarriage

The diagnosis of complete miscarriage can be made when there is a combination of ultrasound scan demonstrating an empty uterine cavity (sometimes

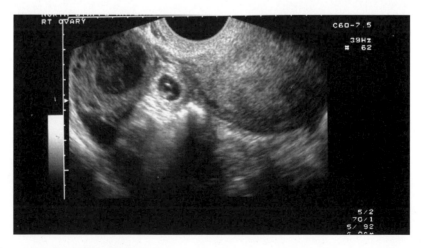

Figure 7.6 Ectopic pregnancy, right adnexa.

termed midline endometrial echo) and a negative pregnancy test (or falling human chorionic gonadotrophin (hCG) levels). Again, caution must be applied as some ectopic pregnancies may present with an empty uterine cavity. Thus it is important to ensure that hormone levels have returned to normal and combine these with the results of the ultrasound scan. A careful history must be taken when a pregnancy test is negative, as women may be incorrectly labelled as having recurrent miscarriages.

Hydatidiform mole

In some cases neoplastic changes may occur in the placental tissue of an anembryonic pregnancy or missed miscarriage. Rarely, a live fetus may also be seen. This can sometimes result in a condition called a hydatidiform mole. The woman usually presents with vaginal bleding, hyperemesis, raised blood pressure and a uterine size larger than her dates. Very rarely a twin gestation may present with one normal fetus and a mole. Moles are benign but may become malignant (choriocarcinoma). The ultrasound diagnosis of a hydatidiform mole is relatively easy and used to be described as a classic 'snowstorm' appearance. Modern ultrasound machines enable visualisation of a placenta that appears vascular and resembles a bunch of grapes. Making this diagnosis is important, as after the mole has been evacuated from the uterus, women with a diagnosed hydatidiform mole require follow-up to exclude subsequent development of choriocarcinoma. It is important that they should be scanned early in their next pregnancy to exclude another mole and they must be re-registered with the trophoblast screening unit at the end of each pregnancy.

MULTIPLE PREGNANCY

Multiple pregnancy accounts for 1 in 80 births and is associated with higher incidences of fetal and maternal morbidity than those involving a single fetus.[12] For the fetus these complications include prematurity, growth difficulties, congenital abnormalities and potential traumatic delivery.[12] For the mother, there is an increased incidence of pre-eclampsia, gestational diabetes, minor ailments of pregnancy and Caesarean section.

Thus, it would seem that for both mother and fetuses, early diagnosis of a multiple pregnancy is desirable. Furthermore, early diagnosis of amnionicity and chorionicity informs the planning of the management of a pregnancy, indicating frequency of scans and biochemical testing, as perinatal mortality is higher for monochorionic and monoamniotic pregnancies, due to the sharing of the circulation in the former, and the sac in the latter.[13]

Zygosity, chorionicity and amnionicity

A single fetus develops from the zygote (fertilisation of an oocyte by one sperm). The zygote divides to produce a clump of cells, the morula, in which a cavity forms, from whence the structure is known as a blastocyst. Occasionally, two separate oocytes are fertilised, which gives rise to 2 zygotes (dizygotic twins). These twins have different genetic patterns and separate sacs and placentae, and are always dichorionic-diamniotic (DC-DA).

Monozygotic twins form from the full division of one zygote, morula or blastocyst. If the morula divides during the first 4 days after implantation, then DC-DA twins result, and the placenta may be separate or fused. If the blastocyst divides between 4 and 8 days after fertilisation, then monochorionic-diamniotic twins result (MC-DA). Vascular connections in the common placenta may result in the complication known as twin-to-twin transfusion syndrome and the subsequent demise of one or both fetuses.

If the blastocyst divides between 8 and 13 days after fertilisation, then monochorionic monoamniotic (MC-MA) twins result. The shared amniotic cavity results in high fetal morbidity and mortality related to entangled umbilical cords and vascular connections.

Figure 7.7 is a diagrammatic representation of the ultrasound appearances of twin pregnancies.

Outcomes

Diagnosis of a multiple pregnancy is confirmed by the visualisation of more than one fetal pole. In the case of twins these should be seen on the screen at the same time.[13] The viability of each should be confirmed by visualising the pulsation of the fetal heart, and gestational age estimated by measuring

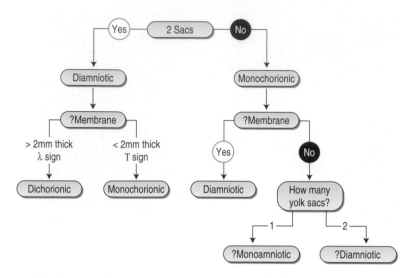

Figure 7.7 Ultrasound indications of amnionicity and chorionicity.

the CRL according to the appropriate criteria. The whole uterus and adnexa should be scanned, longitudinally and transversely, to ensure that no other embryos are missed. Heterotopic pregnancies, although rare, do exist with one intrauterine and one ectopic pregnancy.

Amnionicity and chorionicity

Smith and Smith[13] note that whilst chorionicity can be established at 5 weeks by transvaginal (TV) scan, by visualising the number of gestation sacs present, amnionicity needs to be established later, when the fetal poles can be clearly seen, usually at around 8 weeks by TV scan.

The ultrasound appearances of the intertwin membrane are important in the determination of amnionicity and chorionicity.

MC-MA pregnancies have no intertwin membrane and have a single placenta. The twins will be of the same sex (although this cannot be determined in the first trimester) and there will be intermingling of body parts on the umbilical cords. In extreme cases, where division has occurred very late and is incomplete, then conjoined twins will be seen.

MC-DA twins have a thin membrane (less than 2 mm thick), which is made up of 2 layers of amnion. This membrane inserts in a 'T' configura-

tion into the single placenta. Once again the twins will be of the same sex.

DC-DA twins, who may or may not be of the same sex, have a thick membrane (more than 2 mm thick). This is formed from two layers of amnion and two layers of chorion and the junction with the uterine wall appears wedge shaped, and is often referred to as the 'twin peaks' or 'lambda' sign (see Fig. 7.8)

What do the results mean?

Where there is a diagnosis of MC-MA or MC-DA twins, careful detailed scanning (anatomy survey) of both fetuses should occur, as there is an increased incidence of congenital anomalies in monozygotic twins. In the rare occurrence of conjoined twins (1:50 000–80 000 live births)[14] the extent of joint and organ sharing needs to be assessed and is likely to result in referral to a specialist centre for future management. It should, however, be remembered that dizygotic twins have the same prevalence of congenital anomalies as single pregnancies, and that it is necessary to follow the same protocol for detailed scanning for these pregnancies.

Baseline growth measurements to determine gestational age are important, for the continued assessment of growth and fetal maturity, as intrauterine growth retardation (IUGR) occurs in

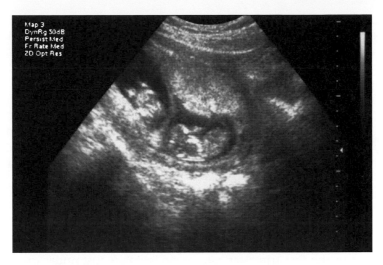

Figure 7.8 Dichorionic diamniotic twins demonstrating the lambda sign.

up to 30% of twin pregnancies.[12] Discordant growth in twins is noted as a result of constitutional variability in dizygotic twins, but may also occur as a result of placental insufficiency, chromosomal abnormality or twin-to-twin transfusion syndrome in monochorionic twins.[12]

Ultrasound features are summarised in Table 7.1 and below:

- All dizygotic twins are DC-DA.
- Where there are separate placentas, then twinning is DC-DA.
- Where fetal sexes differ, twinning is DC-DA.
- If membrane thickness is >2 mm, then probably DC-DA.
- Twin peaks sign denotes DC-DA twinning.

FETAL ANOMALY SCREENING IN EARLY PREGNANCY

Ultrasound is known to be a sensitive tool for the diagnosis of fetal abnormalities in the second trimester. With the advent of high-resolution equipment and transvaginal techniques, it is possible to detect some fetal abnormalities before 13 weeks either because a major abnormality is seen or because there are features suggesting a problem that is confirmed by subsequent tests.

This can be significant for the management of the pregnancy if an abnormality is found and also for the psychological effect on the mother. Early detection of abnormality allows further time for reflection and

Table 7.1 Summary of ultrasound features

Ultrasound features	Zygosity		Amnionicity		Chorionicity	
	MZ	DZ	MA	DA	MC	DC
Different sex possible	N	Y	Y	Y	Y	Y
Two placentas	N	Y	N	Y	N	Y
Membrane >2 mm	N	Y	N	Y	N	Y
Twin peaks (lambda) sign	N	N	N	Y	N	Y

counselling on the options available to the mother. Whilst in the UK there is no upper gestational age for termination of pregnancy for very severe abnormalities, early detection will influence the method of pregnancy termination applied, and enables a choice between surgical and medical management.

Biochemical screening

In parallel with ultrasound studies, routine biochemical tests can also be undertaken in the first trimester to improve detection rates and reduce false positive rates. Ultrasound plays an important role in these tests as it provides essential information about gestational age (see above).

Biochemical screening in the first trimester can be used to enhance the ultrasound information acquired. Biochemical tests in the first trimester can be derived from urine or from serum. The Serum, Urine and Ultrasound Screening Study (SURUSS) reviewed the efficacy, safety and cost effectiveness of a number of tests in combination, in both the first and second trimesters.[15]

In the first trimester the tests include:

- Pregnancy associated plasma protein A (PAPP-A)
- Free hCG (from urine or serum).

The results of the SURUSS study[15] revealed that the most effective and safe method of screening for Down's syndrome in the first trimester should be using a combination of nuchal translucency (see below), free hCG and PAPP-A. Serum markers are discussed in more detail in Chapter 9.

Nuchal translucency

This tool was developed by Snijders et al[16] and calculates the risks of chromosomal abnormality by combining the following parameters:

- Maternal age
- Gestational age and
- Nuchal translucency.

Chitty[17] describes nuchal translucency (NT) as the 'swelling just under the skin at the back of the fetal neck', recognised to be a collection of lymphatic fluid under the skin. The measurement is defined as a sagittal (front to back) measurement between the muscles of the cervical spine and the inner layer of echogenic skin[18] (see Fig. 7.9).

Visualisation is optimum at 10–14 weeks' gestation. An increased NT measurement is associated with chromosomal abnormalities, an increasing risk of structural anomalies (including cardiac defects), neuromuscular problems[19] and a wide range of syndromic problems. The risk of all of these increases as the NT increases from about 2.5 mm upwards.

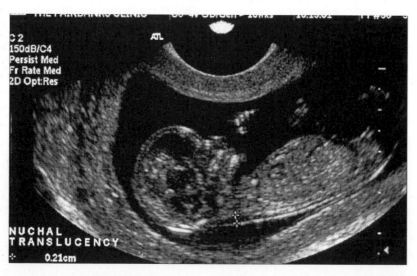

Figure 7.9 Measurement of nuchal translucency.

Criteria for nuchal translucency measurement

- Sagittal section, viewing the length of the spine (see Fig. 7.9).
- Amnion identified separately from the skin surface to ensure measurement accuracy (see Fig. 7.7).
- A standard crown rump length measurement[13] is also calculated to verify gestational age.
- A biparietal diameter (BPD) measurement is also taken where appropriate.
- The heart rate over three cycles is calculated.[20]

With appropriate training and quality assurance mechanisms, nuchal translucency screening is reported to be highly accurate: 80% with 5% false positives.[4] Bahado-Singh et al[3] report that this accuracy can be improved by utilising data of fetal nasal bone measurements. They also report emerging data linking nuchal fluid measurements to the risk of cardiac anomaly, though this still remains a research tool.

ANATOMY/ABNORMALITY SCREENING IN THE FIRST TRIMESTER

During the first trimester of pregnancy some gross structural anomalies can be identified confidently by the well-trained practitioner, using the TV approach. For example, anencephaly (absence of skull and brain tissue) can normally be identified at 10 weeks, after skull ossification has normally occurred. The ultrasound appearances include:

- When trying to obtain a sagittal section the top of the skull will appear small;
- The CRL will be small, but femur length will be appropriate for gestational age;
- A classic 'frog-eyes' appearance of the fetal face.

Knowledge of fetal neural embryology is important to consider to ensure that misdiagnosis does not occur:

- At 7–9 weeks the forebrain appears as a central ventricle.
- At 11–14 weeks the choroid plexus is prominent.

Similarly, cystic hygromas (collections of lymphatic fluid in the posterolateral regions of the neck) of varying severity can be identified from as early as 8 weeks. These fluid collections may be septated or simple and will vary from an increased nuchal thickness (see above) to generalised fetal hydrops.

Eighty percent of fetuses with a cystic hygroma will have an associated chromosomal abnormality and chorion villus sampling (CVS) should be considered (see Ch. 10).

However, caution is needed, as there are pitfalls in diagnosis related to embryological development. For example, at 8–12 weeks the mid gut herniates physiologically into the umbilical cord. Before this period a diagnosis of exomphalos is not reliable, although any herniation noted should not exceed 7 mm.[13]

Where a mother is known to be at high risk of a congenital abnormality (e.g. due to family history or maternal age) then early intervention in the form of transabdominal CVS is offered.

Serum testing can be used in conjunction with nuchal translucency screening to predict the risk of Down's syndrome. However, nuchal translucency scanning requires additional training and skills and is not offered nationally as a routine. Sonographers who have not had specific training, or access to the associated risk calculation software, should not undertake it. If NT screening reveals a high risk of Down's syndrome then it is usual to offer further diagnostic tests, such as either CVS or amniocentesis.

Where there is an increased risk of Down's syndrome indicated, first trimester detailed scanning may offer an enhanced sonographic service, but it should be remembered that 60% of babies with Down's syndrome are structurally normal[20] and that first trimester anomaly scanning is far from routine and requires high-quality ultrasound machines. As machines and training develop further, then it is likely that the role of detailed anomaly scanning in the first trimester will develop.

Finally, it is important when offering any type of screening service, that all staff are trained to support the woman and her partner during this potentially very stressful period of time. The infrastructure of the department must be developed to include counselling and 'quiet' facilities, together with enhanced and sensitive communication methods between all healthcare professionals.

MATERNAL PATHOLOGY

Sometimes during the ultrasound scan maternal pathology is detected. This may be incidental; however, it may have implications for the pregnancy or indeed the mother.

Some types of maternal pathology the sonographer may find are discussed below.

Bicornuate uterus

Bicornuate uterus is a congenital variation which sometimes occurs in females during the embryonic period, which in some women causes the uterus to be doubled.

The appearance of bicornuate uterus varies dependent upon the degree of abnormality. Usually the report should indicate which horn the pregnancy is situated in and if there is any decidual reaction in the other horn that may account for any bleeding. Women with a bicornuate uterus may require surveillance for the growth of the baby and are at increased risk for premature delivery (see Fig. 7.10)

Fibroids

Fibroids are a fairly common finding and are sometimes the cause of pain in pregnancy. They have a variable appearance and this may change during the pregnancy as they can either grow or degenerate. It is important that the sonographer gives an indication of the position of the fibroids. If they

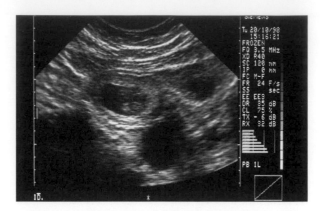

Figure 7.10 Bicornuate uterus with pregnancy in right cornu, decidual reaction in left cornu.

are situated near to the cervix they may affect the delivery of the baby (see Fig. 7.11)

Ovarian cysts

Ovarian cysts are common in pregnancy and may be a result of the corpus luteum. The corpus luteum forms within the follicle after the discharge of the egg for fertilisation. This is an essential endocrine gland in early pregnancy, as it secretes oestrogens and progesterone. It is useful to monitor the size and appearance of ovarian cysts, as they usually disappear if associated with the corpus luteum. Some may persist after the pregnancy or even be more sinister in nature (see Fig. 7.12). Persistent cysts require postnatal evaluation.

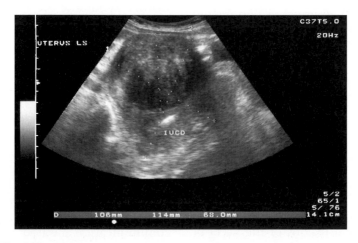

Figure 7.11 IUCD and fibroid in uterus.

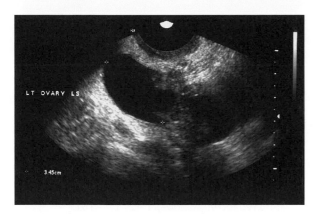

Figure 7.12 Ovarian cyst, left ovary.

Pelvic kidney

This is an incidental normal variant but is important to note as it may be relevant if a Caesarean section needs to be performed.

Intrauterine contraceptive device (IUCD)

The location of an IUCD can be determined and can be important if the clinician is considering removing it during the pregnancy (see Fig. 7.11).

EQUIPMENT SPECIFICATIONS

To undertake ultrasound in the first trimester, a joint report from the Royal College of Obstetricians and Gynaecologists (RCOG) and Royal College of Radiologists (RCR)[9] recommends that both transabdominal (TA) and transvaginal (TV) transducer should be available. The equipment should not be more than 5 years old and should be subject to regular quality assurance checks, including calliper calibration and resolution checks.

In the first trimester it is preferable to perform a TA scan in the first instance and then to proceed to TV scan if adequate detail cannot be obtained to assess the viability of the fetus and obtain an accurate measurement.

TRAINING AND AUDIT

As with any diagnostic procedure, ultrasound should only be undertaken by those who have been suitably trained to do so.[9] Training should include the undertaking of an approved education programme which discusses the principles of ultrasound, leading to an understanding of how the equipment is manipulated to produce high-quality images and consideration of safety issues. Individuals without a recognised qualification (including student sonographers) should always be supervised by qualified staff. For scanning in the first trimester, practitioners should be able to undertake both TV and TA investigations with confidence.[9]

The sonographer should ensure that a locally agreed scheme of work is in place, accept properly delegated responsibility in accordance with local practice, and only perform ultrasound examinations when a valid request card has been received.[21] This is a technology that continually develops and advances in its capability and application; it is therefore essential that practitioners continue to update their knowledge and skills, as well as regularly audit outcomes of their work. It is particularly important where subtle measurements are involved to ensure that measurement criteria are strictly adhered to, such as those for nuchal translucency screening.[4]

CONCLUSION

Bahado-Singh and Chee Cheng[3] comment that it is likely that there will be a shift in the emphasis of obstetric clinical care towards the first trimester and that there will need to be greater research emphasis on the first trimester diagnosis of fetal disorders. We would go further, suggesting that more emphasis be placed on the education and training of sonographers in the anatomy and developmental physiology of the fetus in the first trimester, together with enhancement of interpersonal, communication and counselling skills.

Given that ultrasound plays a pivotal role in the management of pregnancy in the first trimester, it is important that a multidisciplinary communication is maintained, using a client centred approach, to ensure that everyone providing service and care is aware of the woman's particular needs.

As ultrasound machines improve in resolution and ease of operation, it should be remembered that sonographers are highly skilled individuals, trained to utilise the physical properties of ultrasound by manipulating the equipment to produce, interpret and evaluate images that document subtle changes within the fetal and maternal anatomy. The late 1990s demonstrated the dangers of inadequately trained staff utilising the modality.[9] Undoubtedly, the introduction of Early Pregnancy Assessment Units (EPAUs) has improved the care provided to those women experiencing problems in early pregnancy. A study by Wren and Craven in 1999[22] demonstrated that there were both cost and efficiency savings to be made in the provision of an early pregnancy unit. As they comment: 'miscarriage is an emotive subject. Women are extremely distressed when their pregnancy is threatened and demand sensitive and expert medical treatment.'

Key Practice Points

- Early ultrasound dating better predicts expected date of delivery than certain menstrual dates alone.
- A growing number of fetal anomalies can be detected through first trimester ultrasound.
- The first trimester scan can detect maternal pelvic pathology.
- Zygosity and chorionicity should not be confused in multiple pregnancies.
- A raised nuchal translucency measurement can be indicative of a range of chromosomal, genetic and structural problems.
- Ultrasound should only be undertaken by those with adequate training.

Acknowledgements

The authors would like to acknowledge the assistance of Stephen Hodson, Graphic Designer and Sally Edwards, Photographer, Visual Media Department, University of Derby.

References

1. Campbell J, Gilbert WM, Nicolaides KH, Campbell S. Ultrasound screening for spina bifida: cranial and cerebellar signs. Obstetrics and Gynaecology 1987; 70:247–250.
2. Gercosovich EO, Coates TL, Hanson FW, Newberry P. Fetal choroid plexus cysts: maternal, fetal and chromosomal findings in 92 pregnancies. Chicago: Radiological Societies of North America; 1994.
3. Bahado-Singh RO, Chee Cheng CS. First trimester prenatal diagnosis. Current Opinion in Obstetrics and Gynaecology 2004; 16(2):177–181.
4. Pandya PP, Snijders RJM, Johnson SP, et al. Screening for fetal trisomies by maternal age and fetal nuchal translucency thickness at 10 to 14 weeks of gestation. British Journal of Obstetrics and Gynaecology 1995; 102:957–962.
5. Mul T, Mongelli M. Estimating the date of confinement: ultrasonographic biometry versus certain menstrual dates. American Journal of Obstetrics and Gynaecology 1996; 174(1):278–281.
6. Gardosi J, Geirsson R. Routine ultrasound is the method of choice for dating pregnancy. British Journal of Obstetrics and Gynaecology 1998; 105:933–936.
7. Gardosi J. Dating of pregnancy: time to forget the last menstrual period. (Editorial) Ultrasound in Obstetrics and Gynaecology 1997; 9:367–368.
8. West Midlands Perinatal Institute. Perinatal review – induction of labour. dating. 2000. Online. Available: http://www.perinate.org/reviews/iol/iol_dating.htm
9. Royal College of Obstetricians and Gynaecologists and Royal College of Radiologists. Guidance on ultrasound procedures in early pregnancy. Report of the RCR/RCOG Working Party 95(8). London: RCOG/RCR; 1995.
10. CEMACH. Lewis G, ed. Why mothers die 2000–2002. The sixth Report of the Confidential Enquiries into Maternal Deaths in the UK. London: RCOG Press; 2004.
11. Bates J. Practical gynaecological ultrasound. Greenwich: Medical Media; 1997.
12. Sauerbrei EE, Nguyen KT, Nolan RL. A practical guide to ultrasound in obstetrics and gynaecology. 2nd edn. Philadelphia: Lippincott-Raven; 1998: 418.
13. Smith NC, Smith PM. Obstetric ultrasound made easy. Edinburgh: Churchill Livingstone; 2002: 32
14. Campbell GD, Brown SW, Anderson M, Anderson PG. Separation of conjoined twins. Australian &

New Zealand Journal of Surgery 1990;
60(1):59–61.

15. Wald NJ, Rodeck C, Hackshaw AK, et al. First and
second trimester antenatal screening for Down's
syndrome: the results of the Serum, Urine
and Ultrasound Screening Study (SURUSS).
Health Technol Assess 2003; 7(11). Online.
Available: http://www.hta.nhsweb.nhs.uk/
fullmono/mon711.pdf

16. Snijders RJM, Noble P, Sebire N, et al. UK multicentre project on assessment of risk of trisomy 21
by maternal age and fetal nuchal translucency
thickness at 10–14 weeks of gestation. Lancet
1998; 352 (9125):343–346.

17. Pandya PP, Snijders RJM, Johnson SP, et al.
Screening for fetal trisomies by maternal age and
fetal nuchal translucency thickness at 10 to 14
weeks of gestation. International Journal of
Gynecology and Obstetrics 1996; 54(1):86–86(1).

18. Hafner E, Schuchter K, Liebhert E, Philipp K.
Results of routine fetal nuchal translucency

measurement at weeks 10–13 in 4233 unselected
pregnant women. Prenatal Diagnosis 1998;
18(1):29–34.

19. Souka AP, Krampi E, Bakalia S, et al (2001)
Outcome of pregnancy in chromosomally normal
fetuses with increased nuchal translucency in the
first trimester. Ultrasound in Obstetrics and
Gynecology 2001; 18:9–17.

20. Hyett J, Perdu M, Sharland G, et al. Using fetal
nuchal translucency to screen for major congenital cardiac defects at 10–14 weeks of gestation:
population based cohort. British Medical Journal
1999; 318:81–84.

21. United Kingdom Association of Sonographers.
Guidelines for professional working standards in
ultrasound practice. London: UKAS; 2001.

22. Wren J, Craven B. A cost-effectiveness study of
changing medical practice in early pregnancy.
British Journal of Clinical Governance 1999; 4(4):
148–154.

8

The second trimester detailed anomaly scan

Pam Laughna

CHAPTER CONTENTS

INTRODUCTION

The first structural fetal abnormality diagnosed using ultrasound was the demonstration of anencephaly in 1972, followed by the diagnosis of spina bifida 3 years later by the same team.[1,2] Since then, advances in ultrasound have permitted the examination of fetal anatomy to an increasing level of detail and at earlier gestational ages. The list of anomalies which can be detected is lengthy but not all-inclusive. It is important to be aware of the limitations as well as the capabilities of prenatal ultrasound.

Whilst it is possible to gain considerable information regarding fetal anatomy in the first trimester, such ultrasound examinations require high-resolu-tion equipment and a level of expertise which is greater than that offered by most hardworking obstetric ultrasound departments. Taking into account available expertise, equipment, time constraints and detection rates, the Royal College of Obstetricians and Gynaecologists (RCOG) recommend that all pregnant women are offered a routine fetal anomaly scan between 18 and 20 weeks' gestation.[3] This recommendation has since been included in the RCOG/National Institute for Clinical Excellence (NICE) antenatal care guidelines.[4]

The objectives of screening for fetal anomaly include the identification of:

- anomalies that are incompatible with life
- anomalies associated with significant morbidity and long-term disability for the affected individual

125

■ anomalies which may benefit from intrauterine therapy

■ anomalies which may require postnatal investigation or treatment.

The identification of such anomalies during the pregnancy offers the parents the opportunity to have a choice in management options for the pregnancy which may include further investigations (such as karyotyping), a change in the place or mode of delivery, or termination of pregnancy. However, ultrasound in the second trimester may also identify minor structural anomalies which in themselves may not be significant but the identification of which may cause considerable anxiety in the parents.

There is considerable debate as to whether or not routine anomaly scans have led to an improvement in pregnancy outcome. The Routine Antenatal Diagnostic Imaging with Ultrasound RADIUS study[5] failed to demonstrate any significant benefit in terms of outcome, although the detection rate of anomalies was very low (16 % overall).[6] However, European experience has demonstrated an effect on perinatal mortality secondary to fetal anomaly, probably through termination of pregnancy.[7,8] The sensitivity of routine fetal anomaly scans in the screening for fetal abnormality in the UK varies, depending on the severity of the anomaly and the experience of the sonographer. Detection rates for anencephaly, for example, exceed 99% whereas major cardiac malformations are detected with a sensitivity which varies from 4 to 77%.

Although the benefits to perinatal mortality may be secondary to a shift in the pregnancy loss to the second trimester, by virtue of termination of pregnancy, there are data to suggest that perinatal outcome is improved following prenatal diagnosis of some congenital anomalies. This is particularly relevant for cardiac anomalies[9] and anomalies which require early postnatal surgical correction, e.g. gastroschisis.

In addition to screening for structural malformations, the second trimester scan offers an opportunity for dating the pregnancy with an accuracy of within 14 days either side of the estimated date of delivery. Therefore, in obstetric units which can only offer one routine scan during pregnancy, the second trimester scan between 18 and 20 weeks provides the best compromise. Current recommendation from both NICE and the National Screening Committee in the United Kingdom is that women are offered both a dating scan before 13 weeks and an anomaly scan.

CONDUCT OF THE SCAN

The fetal anomaly scan should be performed in a suitable scan room offering privacy to the mother. It is common practice to allow an accompanying person to witness the scan, usually the partner or relative of the mother. It is important that mothers are aware of the purpose of the scan, i.e:

■ to confirm that the pregnancy is ongoing
■ to confirm dates or normal growth (if a dating scan has been performed)
■ to exclude multiple pregnancy (if no dating scan has been performed)
■ to exclude fetal abnormality
■ to identify placental position.

Whilst it is not currently universal practice to obtain written consent for ultrasound scans in pregnancy, this is becoming more common. It is recommended that all women receive written information about the nature and purpose of the scan in advance of the scan appointment.[10] It is important that the mother realise that the scan is not compulsory and the decision not to have one performed must be respected. The information given, be it written or oral, should include information about the limitations of the scan so that mothers are aware that not all congenital malformations can be detected on routine ultrasonography. Similarly, if certain structures are not routinely visualised, or cannot be visualised in a particular fetus, the mother should be aware of this.

The scan department should have the facility to offer a quiet room which may be used for counselling if an abnormality is discovered.

Ideally, a printed report is issued although many units rely on handwritten reports. The use of an ultrasound or fetal medicine database enhances audit activity, which is an integral part of good clinical practice. Those involved in prenatal ultrasound should be encouraged to attend multidisciplinary meetings such as perinatal mortality or dysmorphology meetings in order to facilitate audit and continuing education.

The sonographer should exclude multiple pregnancy and establish that the fetus is alive before demonstrating the fetus and fetal heart activity briefly to the mother. The scan is then performed in a systematic way, initially identifying fetal lie within the uterus, placental position and an assessment of liquor volume before commencing the fetal measurements. Demonstration of the fetus to the mother has been shown to have a positive effect on bonding.

The exact detail in which the fetal anatomy is examined will depend upon local practice and the sonographer's expertise. It is recommended that all obstetric units that offer a routine fetal anomaly scan have an agreed protocol for the scan. It is common practice to produce a checklist on which the final report of the scan is based. Not only does this provide an *aide mémoire* for the sonographers, it also allows the mother to see which anatomy has been examined.

FETAL BIOMETRY

Whilst the majority of women in the UK have a dating scan performed during the first 14 weeks of pregnancy, fetal biometry before 24 weeks offers a satisfactory and reliable method of dating a pregnancy with an error of 14 days either side of the expected date of delivery. The measurements of choice at this stage of pregnancy are the biparietal diameter (BPD) and femur length (FL).[11] In order to use such measurements for dating, it is essential that adequate images be obtained. It is good practice to measure both. If there is agreement between the gestational age assessment of the BPD and FL measurements, and this differs from the menstrual dates by more than 7 days, the ultrasonic assessment of gestational age should be adopted and the menstrual dates discarded. If the assessments of gestational age derived from the BPD and FL differ from one another by more than 7 days, then the possibility of a fetal abnormality should be considered, e.g. short limbed dwarfism.

It is good practice to confirm normal fetal growth when second trimester scan measurements are used to date a pregnancy by repeating the scan 2–4 weeks later.

In addition to BPD and FL, the head circumference (HC) and abdominal circumference (AC) should be measured at the time of the routine scan. Whilst not essential for dating purposes, they provide a baseline against which further scans may be compared at later gestations.

FETAL ANATOMY

Central nervous system

The fetal skull, brain and spine are examined. The skull should have normal ossification and be of an oval shape. Intracranial structures are identified, including the midline, cavum septum pellucidum, cerebellum and lateral ventricles. The spine should be examined along its length in transverse and sagittal planes.

Neural tube defects are common. Anencephaly has a high detection rate (approaching 100%) with between 69% and 100% of cases of spina bifida (see Fig. 1) being detected.

Thorax

The principle view obtained of the thorax is at the level of the heart, which should occupy approximately one-third of the area, with its apex to the left side. The thoracic size should be seen to be normal.

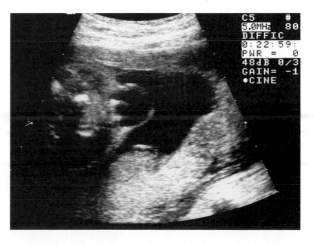

Figure 8.1 Transverse section of lumbar meningomyelocoele.

Heart

Congenital abnormalities of the heart are common, with an incidence of approximately 8 per 1000. However, many anomalies cannot be detected before birth, e.g. atrial septal defects (ASD) and patent ductus arteriosus (PDA) because of the differences between the fetal and postnatal circulations. Screening for congenital heart disease may either be based on the four chamber view of the heart, or incorporate the great vessels (aorta and pulmonary artery). Not all major abnormalities will be apparent on the four chamber view, e.g. tetralogy of Fallot, and this view alone will limit the detection rate of major anomalies to between 25% and 50%. The addition of the great vessels increases the detection rate to between 60% and 75%.

Screening for congenital heart disease has been disappointing in its effectiveness, but educational programmes such as that initiated by Guy's Hospital in the 1980s and continued by charities such as ECHO (Effective Cardiac Health in Obstetrics, *www.echocharity.org.uk*) have led to improvements. Sonographers require additional training to be able to examine both the four chamber view and the great vessels, and local practice will reflect the level of training which is available.

Whilst all organ systems can show developmental changes during gestation such that anomalies become more apparent as the pregnancy progresses, this is particularly pertinent in screening for congenital heart disease. Rhythm disturbances (such as supraventricular tachycardias) rarely present before the third trimester and are often associated with a structurally normal heart.

Abdomen

It is important to confirm the integrity of the anterior abdominal wall by examining the cord insertion, as well as examining the intra-abdominal organs. The fetal stomach should be seen as a fluid-filled structure below the diaphragm and under the fetal heart. The fetal bowel is usually of a similar echolucency to fetal lung and dilatation is rarely seen before the third trimester.

Bowel atresias, including duodenal atresia, present as dilated proximal bowel but are rarely apparent at the time of the routine fetal anomaly scan.

Urogenital tract

The fetal kidneys are identified lying either side of the spine, and normal renal architecture can be identified. The fetal bladder is an echofree structure lying within the fetal pelvis with the umbilical arteries running either side. Normal ureters are not visible.

The renal tract in the fetus is dynamic, i.e. the fetus is producing urine. It is therefore possible for appearances to change during a scan, i.e. for a bladder to fill and empty. Urinary tract obstructions can be present from early in development, e.g. urethral atresia, or present later in gestation, e.g. pelviureteric junction obstruction. Some obstructive lesions may resolve, e.g. posterior urethral valves. Therefore, the urinary tract may demonstrate marked differences in appearance with advancing gestation.

The external genitalia can be visualised at the fetal anomaly scan. Absence of male genitalia does not confirm female sex, and fetal sexing can only be done by positive identification of either male or female external genitalia. Each unit has its own policy regarding fetal sexing, with opinion being divided as to whether or not parents should be informed of the fetal sex. Examination of the external genitalia does not form part of the recommended protocol for routine anomaly scan.[10]

Skeleton and extremities

The long bones of the limbs should be examined to confirm shape and the presence of three long bones in each of the four limbs. The presence and attitude of the hands and feet can also be examined. It is not routine to count the number of digits. Whilst the femur is the long bone which is routinely measured to assess gestational age and fetal growth, if the femur length is discordant with other biometry, it is possible to measure the other long bones to assess the possibility of a skeletal dysplasia.

The ossification of the skeleton is assessed subjectively. Disorders of ossification are rare, but if there is an abnormality it is usually apparent at the time of the anomaly scan.

Face

The orbits, nose, lips and profile can be examined (see Fig. 8.2), although this does not form part of many routine scans.

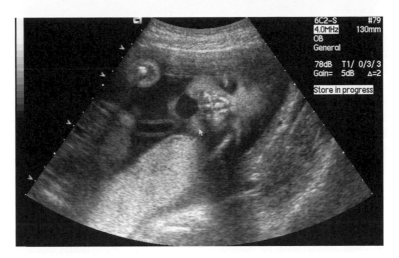

Figure 8.2 Fetal face with mouth open.

PLACENTA AND AMNIOTIC FLUID VOLUME

In addition to assessing fetal viability, size and anatomy, the anomaly scan provides an opportunity to examine the placental site and the liquor volume. The placental site is usually described in broad terms, i.e. anterior or posterior, low or not low. If the placenta is seen to encroach upon or cover the internal cervical os, it is advisable to re-examine the placental site at 34–36 weeks' gestation when the lower segment of the uterus will have formed.

By the time of the routine anomaly scan, the liquor volume is mostly composed of fetal urine. Abnormalities of the renal tract may lead to a reduction or absence of amniotic fluid. Oligohydramnios or anhydramnios may make visualisation of the fetal anatomy very difficult. An excessive amniotic fluid volume is rarely found at this gestation, being more common towards the end of the second trimester or during the third.

FACTORS AFFECTING THE LIMITATIONS OF ULTRASOUND

It is important to realise the second trimester ultrasound is limited in its ability to detect certain abnormalities and that many factors can limit this further. Such factors include:

- maternal obesity
- abdominal scarring
- fetal lie and position
- oligohydramnios or anhydramnios
- multiple pregnancy.

The ability to examine fetal anatomy in detail is also limited by the quality of the ultrasound equipment available. All modern ultrasound equipment has sufficiently high resolution to be appropriate for obstetric examinations, as long as the equipment is well maintained with appropriate transducers. The RCOG recommend that equipment should be replaced every 5 years unless it is possible to upgrade the system, which is possible on many modern top-range scanners.

Most ultrasound machines today will be equipped with a curvilinear transducer of variable frequency. The frequency of ultrasound dictates the resolution (the higher the frequency, the better the resolution) and the penetration (the lower the frequency, the greater the depth of penetration). In order to obtain a high-resolution image in pregnancy, frequencies of 3–6 MHz are used for second trimester work and 2–4 MHz for the third trimester, when the depth of penetration required is greater because of the size of the uterus and its contents. The advent of multifrequency transducers (4–6 MHz on one transducer) has enabled units to reduce the number of transducers that they need, as a single transducer will often be adequate for all scans. However, in very obese women, it may be necessary to use a lower frequency in order to achieve adequate visualisation.

If abdominal wall scarring is present, it is difficult to achieve good views through the scar tissue which, if extensive, may significantly limit the quality of the scan.

Fetal lie and position may make adequate examination impossible. If the mother is encouraged to walk around for a few minutes, the fetus will often move into another position. Similarly, filling and/or emptying the mother's urinary bladder may help. It may be impossible to complete the scan on a single occasion and then the mother should be recalled between 1 and 2 weeks later so that the scan may be finished. It is important to reassure the mother in such cases that no problem has been identified, but that the fetal position has precluded a complete examination. In some cases, use of the transvaginal transducer may assist.

When difficulty is experienced in achieving a complete examination, this should be recorded as well as the reason why. Units will have their own policy about recalling women if certain anatomical structures have not been fully examined, e.g. most hospitals will recall a woman in whom the fetal spine has not been clearly visualised, but may not recall if one kidney was not seen as long as the bladder, other kidney and liquor volume were seen to be normal.

Sometimes anomalies develop later in pregnancy than the time of the anomaly scan and thus will not be detected unless further scans are performed for any reason and anatomy is reassessed.

COMMON ABNORMALITIES DIAGNOSED ON THE ROUTINE SCAN

Abnormalities which can be detected on routine scan can be divided into major and minor anomalies. Major anomalies are those which pose a risk to the life of the fetus, either in utero or in the postnatal period. They may be associated with neuro developmental problems or require surgical correction after delivery. Minor anomalies may require treatment after birth, but will not pose a risk to the life or development of the affected individual. Both major and minor anomalies can be associated with other problems such as abnormal chromosomes or genetic syndromes.

Table 8.1 illustrates common major abnormalities, their approximate frequencies and associated

Table 8.1 **Common major malformations**

Anomaly	Incidence (per 1000 births)	Associated anomalies
Spina bifida	2–4	Trisomy 13, trisomy 18, sodium valproate therapy
Anencephaly	2–4	Trisomy 13, trisomy 18
Cleft lip	1–2	Cleft palate, trisomy 13,18 and 21
Congenital heart disease	8	Aneuploidy, maternal diabetes
Diaphragmatic hernia	0.3–0.5	Aneuploidy, neural tube defects, exomphalos, duodenal atresia, renal anomalies, congenital heart defects
Exomphalos	0.2	Trisomy 13, trisomy 18, Bechwith Wiedeman syndrome, congenital heart defects, neural tube defects
Gastroschisis	0.1	Maternal cocaine use
Duodenal atresia	0.1	Trisomy 21
Renal agenesis	0.1–0.3	Fraser syndrome, VATER syndrome, congenital heart defects, gastrointestinal anomalies
Bladder outflow obstruction	0.01	Posterior urethral valves

anomalies. Such associated anomalies often relate to common embryological origins (e.g. they may all arise from the same embryological layer such as the mesoderm). Recognised patterns of anomalies may be grouped together as syndromes, e.g. VATER (Vertebral anomalies, Anal atresia, TracheooEsophageal fistula, Renal anomalies). When an anomaly is detected, it is important to conduct a thorough search for any additional abnormality.

Table 8.2 illustrates common minor anomalies and associations. Many minor anomalies are described as markers for chromosomal abnormalities. It is extremely rare for an isolated minor anomaly to be an indication of aneuploidy, but the risks increase when two or more markers are identified.

WHAT HAPPENS WHEN AN ABNORMALITY IS SEEN OR SUSPECTED?

The sonographers will often be in a position to make a firm diagnosis when an anomaly is seen, e.g. spina bifida, exomphalos. However, in many cases the sonographers will recognise that the appearances are not normal but may not be able to make a firm diagnosis. In common with midwives, obstetric sonographers are trained to confirm normality and recognise what is not normal, or does not appear to be, without the necessity to make a firm diagnosis each time. It is often beyond their expertise and experience to make a firm diagnosis. In these circumstances, a repeat ultrasound by a more experienced person (usually a consultant) will be offered. This may require referral to another centre. This period of uncertainty can be distressing and in general, fetal medicine units will endeavour to offer this scan with minimal delay.

Further management may include:

- further ultrasound with obstetrician or radiologist to confirm diagnosis
- referral to a regional fetal medicine unit
- discussion about further investigations such as karyotyping
- management options such as termination of pregnancy (if appropriate), delivery at a tertiary referral unit, etc.

It is important that the mother is given accurate information about any problems that are identified. This inevitably causes upset and anxiety, and it is essential to allow the parents sufficient time to consider the implications of any diagnosis, not only for the affected baby but also for the existing family. Whilst it is important not to introduce undue delay in establishing a suitable plan of management, it is also necessary to avoid unseemly hurry. The delay of 24 hours between initial diagnosis and confirmation and discussion of further investigations with subsequent options is usually beneficial to the parents as they have a chance to discuss the implications in their own home and in their own time.

If the anomaly is one which is associated with aneuploidy, discussion about karyotyping should take place. Options will usually include amniocentesis (which can normally be performed locally), chorionic villus sampling or fetal blood sampling, both of which may require referral to the local fetal medicine unit. It is necessary to be aware that if karyotyping is left until after delivery if the pregnancy is terminated, e.g. on products of conception, the chance of obtaining a karyotype is reduced to approximately 70%.[12]

SAFETY OF ULTRASOUND

Ultrasound has now been applied in pregnancy for more than one generation. Women who were

Table 8.2 Common minor anomalies

Minor anomaly	Association	Risk of aneuploidy (if isolated)
Choroid plexus cysts	Trisomy 13 and 18	1.5 × a priori risk
Renal pelvis dilatation	Trisomy 13, 18, 21	1.5 × a priori risk
Echogenic bowel	Trisomy 21, cystic fibrosis	5.5 × a priori risk
Single umbilical artery	Trisomy 21, IUGR	1.5 × a priori risk
Short femur	Trisomy 21	2.5 × a priori risk

themselves scanned when fetuses are now undergoing pregnancy. Thus, if there was any significant adverse effect of ultrasound on the developing fetus and germ cells, it should now be becoming apparent. No such harmful effects have been shown.

Confirmation of safety is virtually impossible for any technology applied to human pregnancy. Ultrasound has the potential to cause harm as it is a form of energy. Attempts to assess the safety of ultrasound have been directed in two areas:

- epidemiological evidence from populations that have been exposed
- laboratory experiments of the interactions of ultrasound with biological materials.

Both methods have limitations, but there is now a reasonable literature addressing this important issue.

In 1988, the American Institute for Ultrasound in Medicine and Biology (AIUM) stated that:

> No confirmed biological effects in patients or operators caused by exposures at intensities typical of the present diagnostic ultrasound instruments have ever been reported. Although the possibility exists that problems may arise in the future, current data indicate the benefits from the approved use of ultrasound outweigh the risks—if any—that may be present.

It is, however, important to remember that ultrasound has the potential to cause harm and thus the ALAR principle (As Low As Reasonably Attainable) should be applied to ultrasound exposure in pregnancy. Any scan performed should have a specific purpose with the result being necessary for the clinical management of the pregnancy.

The addition of Doppler ultrasound to examine the fetal circulation increases the energy output of ultrasound, and the British Medical Ultrasound Society in 1991 stated:

In pulsed Doppler examinations

- particular care should be taken in obstetric applications
- keep negative pressure to a minimum
- avoid tissue/bone interfaces
- beware patients with elevated temperatures.

However, epidemiologists have looked at various outcome measures to assess the safety of obstetric ultrasound.

Childhood cancer

No association has been found between exposure to ultrasound and the development of childhood cancers, although the data are old (30 years).

Dyslexia

A large Norwegian study[13] found no correlation between *in utero* exposure to ultrasound and dyslexia, although an earlier smaller study had suggested that there was an association. This has not been confirmed in subsequent studies.

Non-right handedness

The same study in Norway did find a correlation between non-right handedness and fetal exposure to ultrasound, although subsequent studies by the same group[14] have not confirmed this.

Delayed speech development

An early Canadian study suggested an association between fetal exposure to ultrasound and delayed speech, but this has not been confirmed in larger studies.

Low birth weight

One problem with any relationship between ultrasound and low birth weight is that fetuses identified before birth as having a reduced growth velocity have a greater exposure to ultrasound. However, a review of the literature in 1995 did not find a significant relationship and studies looking at size at 1 year of age similarly fail to demonstrate any association.

In summary, therefore, no adverse consequences to the individual related to prenatal exposure to ultrasound have been demonstrated in large epidemiological studies.

CONCLUSION

On current evidence, routine fetal anomaly scans in the second trimester have improved perinatal mortality figures secondary to congenital malformation and have led to some improvements in morbidity. There is also benefit in terms of maternal satisfaction and bonding. When an anomaly is detected, parents appreciate the advantages of being forewarned prior to the birth, so that they know what to expect particularly if postnatal treatment is required. No harmful effects of ultrasound on the developing fetus have been established.

When an anomaly is detected, further investigations may be appropriate in order to gain the maximum amount of information which can be used to plan the subsequent management.

References

1. Campbell S, Johnstone F, et al. Anencephaly: early ultrasonic diagnosis and active management. Lancet 1972; 2:1226–1227.
2. Campbell S, Pryse-Davies J, et al. Ultrasound in the diagnosis of spina bifida. Lancet 1975; 1: 1065–1068.
3. RCOG. Ultrasound screening for fetal abnormalities. Report of the RCOG Working Party. London: Royal College of Obstetricians and Gynaecologists; 1997.
4. RCOG, NICE. Antenatal care: routine care for the healthy pregnant woman. Clinical guideline. London: Royal College of Obstetricians and Gynaecologists, National Institute for Clinical Excellence; 2003; 72–74.
5. Ewigman B, Crane J, et al. Effect of prenatal ultrasound screening on perinatal outcome. RADIUS Study Group. N Engl J Med 1993; 329:821–827.
6. Crane J, LeFevre M, et al. A randomized trial of prenatal ultrasonographic screening: impact on the detection, management and outcome of the anomalous fetus. Am J Obstet Gynecol 1994; 171:392–399.
7. Saari-Kemppainen A, Karjalainen O, et al. Ultrasound screening and perinatal mortality: controlled trial of one-stage screening in pregnancy. Lancet 1990; 336:387–391.
8. Bucher H, Schmidt J. Does routine ultrasound scanning improve the outcome of pregnancy? Meta-analysis of various outcomes. BMJ 1993; 307:13–18.
9. Yates R. The influence of prenatal diagnosis on postnatal outcome in patients with structural congenital heart disease. Prenat Diagn 2004; 24:1143–1149.
10. RCOG. Routine ultrasound screening in pregnancy. Protocols, standards and training. London: Royal College of Obstetricians and Gynaecologists; 2000.
11. British Medical Ultrasound Society. Clinical applications of ultrasonic fetal measurements: Fetal Measurements Working Party Report. London: British Institute of Radiology; 1990.
12. Kyle P, Sepulveda W, et al. High failure rate of postmortem karyotyping after termination for fetal abnormality. Obstet Gynecol 1996; 88:859–862.
13. Salvesen KA, Bakketeig LS, Feik-nes SH, et al. Routine ultrasonography in utero and school performance at age 8–9 years Lancet Jan 11 1992; 339 (8785):85–89.
14. Salvesen KA, Feik-nes SH. Is ultrasound normal? A review of epidemiological studies of human exposure to ultrasound. Ultrasound Obstet Gynecol Oct 1995; 6:293–298.

9

Biochemical markers in Down's syndrome screening

Pat Ward

INTRODUCTION

Screening for Down's syndrome during pregnancy is undertaken using a variety of techniques and technologies. Screening tests vary, e.g. biochemical analysis, ultrasound measurement, assessment of age, and therefore the given risk involved varies. Diagnostic testing usually utilises either amniocentesis or chorionic villus sampling. As with any screening programme the screening test is just that, a screening test and not a diagnostic test. Therefore screening for Down's syndrome is a two step process: first, screening to identify those women who are at higher risk, and then a diagnostic test to confirm the status of the screening result. This is the same principle for any screening programme.

THE DEVELOPMENT OF BIOCHEMICAL SCREENING

Although the classification of the syndrome was made in 1864 by Dr John Langdon Down,[1] it wasn't until 1933 that the association of maternal age and the increased risk of having a child with Down's syndrome was first realised. Following the discovery of the ability to use the karyotype to diagnose a person with Down's syndrome, and using the knowledge that Down's syndrome occurred in pregnancies of older women, the first analyses of amniotic fluid (prenatal diagnosis) took place in 1968.[2] This allowed older women to be offered prenatal diagnosis with age being the initial screening tool and amniocentesis the diagnostic tool. The development of these technologies and the impact on how women experience pregnancy is discussed in more detail in Chapter 1.

However, this service was limited to those hospitals who were able to offer and fund it. It was usually on a limited basis and dependent on clinical availability and experience of the obstetrician to perform the amniocentesis. In 1984, with the first realisation that a low alpha-fetoprotein (AFP) was associated with Down's syndrome, work commenced concentrating on biochemical markers in the maternal blood which would give the ability to screen on a larger population scale than could be offered with diagnostic services.[3]

The first discovery that AFP would be helpful in screening was associated with Edwards syndrome, when a patient noted to her clinician that she had a low level of AFP after giving birth to a child with Edwards syndrome. Research was soon expanded to assess its capability for Down's syndrome, the most common chromosomal abnormality found at birth.

Chromosomes contain all genetic material which codes for our physical and intellectual capabilities. The normal complement is 46 chromosomes arranged in 23 pairs, each pair containing a chromosome from each parent. In a trisomic condition the person has an extra chromosome. For instance, people with Down's syndrome have an extra chromosome number 21 (i.e. trisomy 21). Edwards syndrome (trisomy 18) occurs when there is an additional chromosome 18. This gives extra genetic material and disrupts the normal DNA processes which form the basis of 'normal' levels of intellectual and physical developments in a person. A karyotype is the name given to describe the complement of chromosomes which each person has in their cells.

Continuation of work in the biochemistry research field during the mid to late 1980s gave the further discovery that human chorionic gonadotrophin (hCG) was raised in Down's syndrome pregnancies, followed by the ability to use estriol (uE3) as a screening marker in the late 1980s and early 1990s. Estriol is normally low in Down's syndrome pregnancies.[4] All these markers, their biochemistry background and use will be discussed in this chapter.

Other markers, such as the measurement of the nuchal translucency by ultrasound scanning techniques, really gained popularity during the early to mid 1990s when evidence on their utility became more certain. Nuchal translucency scanning measured the depth of skin and subcutaneous fluid at the nape of the neck in a fetus. The larger the measurement the greater the risk of the fetus being affected with Down's syndrome.[5] This is discussed in more detail in Chapter 7. These markers have remained for some time the most advanced markers in screening for Down's syndrome and are the most commonly used today. However, as is discussed later in the chapter, there are new markers and strategies which may eventually supersede the detection rates of the original and conventional ones.

It is extensively published that the risk of having a child with Down's syndrome increases with maternal age[6] (see Table 9.1). The prevalence is around 1 in 800 births and therefore if around 3000 women a year were screened one would expect an average of four Down's syndrome pregnancies to be born in that group. The increase in risk is correlated to age and this is also the same for other chromosomal trisomies such as Edwards syndrome (trisomy 18) and Patau's syndrome (trisomy13), although the prevalence at birth for these conditions is lower, at 1 in 1500 and 1 in 3000 respectively.

It must be remembered that trisomy 21 is not the most common chromosome condition occurring but the one in which the fetus will more likely survive to term. Others such as trisomy 15 and 16 will be more common but it is unlikely that a fetus with these conditions will survive beyond the second trimester of pregnancy.

The National Down's Syndrome Cytogenetics Register (NDSCR) collects statistics on the prevalence and results of screening modalities. The average age of a woman conceiving has increased by 2 years since 1989. Therefore the prevalence of Down's syndrome in the population has increased by this margin. To try and explain this in relation to the effect on a local screening programme, it is well known that if a screened population was on average older than expected then more Down's syndrome pregnancies would occur and therefore more Down's affected pregnancies should be detected by the screening test. This is one of the reasons why some local screening programmes may have a better detection rate than others if their pregnant population is on average older than another.

Table 9.1 The risk of having a pregnancy affected by Down's syndrome

Age of a woman in years	Risk (chance) of having an affected baby
20	1:1500
22	1:1450
24	1:1400
26	1:1250
28	1:1100
30	1:900
32	1:650
34	1:450
36	1:280
38	1:160
40	1:100
42	1:55
44	1:30

A recent publication shows this clearly using retrospective data of over 600 000 pregnancies and 1000 Down's-syndrome-affected pregnancies.[7] The screened population was divided into age groups of 5 years and the detection and false-positive rates (FPR) calculated for those respective groups. The older age groups have better detection rates but certainly higher FPRs. It also clearly showed that the detection rates for pregnant women over 40 years of age is almost 100% with an FPR of around 50%. Therefore the argument that all women should be offered a diagnostic test in preference to a screening test is no longer acceptable as a screening policy.

TIMING OF THE TEST

Screening for Down's syndrome and the use of biochemical and ultrasound markers can only be used at certain times during the gestation. Screening cannot take place before 10 weeks of pregnancy as the proteins and hormones measured are not sufficiently stable or consistent in the maternal system to be measured accurately. A nuchal translucency ultrasound measurement should not be performed either before 11 weeks, as it cannot be accurately measured.

It is important to remember that Down's syndrome screening should take place before 20 weeks of pregnancy, this is to allow for diagnostic techniques to be implemented and give an adequate time window for decisions around the management of the pregnancy to take place as early as possible. Women should be encouraged to decide upon their choices as early as possible in the pregnancy and should have sufficient time to make an informed decision with their partner. It is possible to screen up until 23 weeks of pregnancy using biochemical and ultrasound markers but it is not ideal to do so. If a woman would like this to occur, it should be discussed with local clinicians and biochemistry departments to assess the pathways of clinical management following the result if an affected pregnancy was found and termination of the pregnancy was requested.

BIOCHEMICAL MARKERS

A chemical substance is described in the dictionary as a substance produced by a living organism or involving chemical processes in a living organism. In screening for Down's syndrome and fetal anomalies there are a variety of biochemical markers which can be used. When biochemists use the word 'marker' it refers to a particular hormone or protein and often can be used interchangeably with analyte. However, analyte is particular to biochemistry. When we discuss markers in ultrasound it means a measurement taken or an anatomical variant noted, such as a large nuchal translucency measurement or the absence of nasal bone.

There has been a proliferation of markers discovered since the realisation in 1984 that AFP levels were low in trisomic pregnancies. They have been specifically researched and designed for their use within the Down's syndrome screening programme and each could be used individually, to indicate a risk, or, more effectively, they could be used in a combined manner to give a better indication of risk. The different biochemical markers in common use today are human chorionic gonadotrophin (hCG), unconjugated estriol (uE3), alphafetoprotein (AFP) and inhibin-A. These are second trimester markers, i.e. they should only be used for screening for Down's syndrome from 14 weeks onwards, except hCG.

Pregnancy associated plasma protein A (PAPP-A), which is a first trimester marker, can be used from 10–14 weeks of pregnancy. It can also be used with hCG, which is the only marker that can be useful throughout both the first and second trimesters of pregnancy. The effectiveness of the biochemistry and ultrasound markers are demonstrated in the Health and Technology Assessment (HTA) report[8] and shown in Table 9.2.

hCG

All of the markers originate from various places in the maternal and fetal system. hCG originates from the placenta and can be divided into three different types: total, intact and free beta. The total hCG is a measurement of the whole of the hCG molecule, (alpha and beta); the free bhCG is one particular part of the beta hCG; and the intact measures the whole of the beta molecule only. The alpha hCG is part of a subunit. This has been used in some research areas to see if it improves the detection rate for Down's syndrome screening but has now been discarded in favour of free beta hCG. Therefore, when discussing screening and screening markers, it is important to ensure that you know which type of hCG is being used within your programme. Most commonly free beta hCG is the one favoured and this is used both in the first trimester and second trimester. All of these markers have different screening detection rates.

AFP

AFP is a product of the yolk sac and fetal liver. The fetus excretes a large amount of AFP into the amniotic fluid and therefore one of the important points to remember is that if a diagnostic procedure has been performed before the AFP blood serum is taken, then the AFP will be raised considerably and give a false result. This is due to leakage of the amniotic fluid into the maternal system causing a raised AFP. When undertaking screening the blood should be taken before any diagnostic techniques have been performed.

Table 9.2 **Biochemical markers for Down's syndrome**

Type of marker	Most effective
PAPP-A	10–14 weeks
hCG (free bhCG used in both trimesters, total, intact bhCG in second)	10–22 weeks
Alpha hCG	No longer used
uE3	14–22 weeks
AFP	15–20 weeks
Inhibin-A	15–20 weeks

AFP and structural anomalies

AFP is also a screening tool for neural tube defects (NTDs) (spina bifida and anencephaly, most commonly) and as such is a useful marker for other conditions. However, unlike Down's syndrome screening, when a low AFP indicates increased risk for Down's syndrome, in screening for NTDs the level of AFP is much higher than expected. In most units it is the policy to investigate any levels over 2.5 multiples of the median (MOM). This will be explained later in the chapter. The diagnostic tool of choice, following the discovery of a raised AFP, is a detailed ultrasound scan to look for any structural signs of NTD. It should also be remembered that a raised AFP can also be a sign of other structural anomalies such as gastrochisis and exomphalos. Exomphalos is associated with trisomy 13 and therefore it is usual practice to offer a diagnostic test to find out the karyotype status of the pregnancy in this situation. These two conditions are major defects of the abdominal wall and can be quite clearly seen on an ultrasound scan.

UE3

Unconjugated estriol is a product of the adrenal glands of fetus. In a Down's syndrome pregnancy the level is usually lowered.

PAPP-A

PAPP-A is a product of the placenta and is most effective for Down's syndrome screening in the first trimester, when it is lower than normal. In Down's syndrome screening the most effective time to use PAPP-A is at 10 weeks' gestation.

Inhibin-A

Inhibin A is a biochemistry marker used mainly in the second trimester. The most important thing to remember is that the levels are affected by smoking, which can cause up to a 47% difference from the expected level. It is therefore important that, if incorporating inhibin A as part of your screening programme, the smoking status of women should be sought and documented on the request form.[9] The levels are not dependent upon the number of cigarettes that are smoked, purely on the fact that the woman smokes.

ASSESSMENT OF BIOCHEMICAL LEVELS

The expected levels of all hormones and proteins are well documented and can be easily measured in a laboratory. Some, such as hCG and inhibin-A, are quite high during the initial establishment of the pregnancy, then decrease as other hormones, such as AFP and estriol, take over the continuation of the pregnancy. Hormone levels become more stable during the late second trimester, but at this point it is too late to screen because of the late time window for a termination of pregnancy. It is vitally important that the correct date of the pregnancy is known. If the date of the pregnancy is given wrongly, the laboratory will compare the level found in the maternal blood with the wrong point on the chart and therefore misinterpret the level, leading to an incorrect result. Establishing the correct gestational date cannot be emphasised too much in a screening programme such as this.

To explain this further, the biochemical markers are present in the maternal blood in differing quantities. During pregnancy the levels also rise and fall with gestational age of the pregnancy. Establishing levels of hormones and proteins in a patient's blood to assess their risk of a disease is the everyday work of the biochemistry department. The way that levels rise and fall during pregnancy can be seen in Figure 9.1.

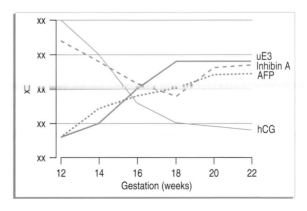

Figure 9.1 Changes in levels of biochemical markers during the first trimester of pregnancy.

In Down's syndrome screening, the normal levels are well established. The method for understanding what the normal level should be is to analyse all samples of blood that are taken from a pregnant population for screening and plot them. By doing this the expected level for each week of screening can be seen. This forms the baseline for other pregnancies to be measured against and the levels of screening tests can be added into the data to refine it even more. Eventually the laboratory will establish a large data set of the levels of the markers for each week and therefore understand what the norm should be. It is evident that a laboratory undertaking a large volume of work will therefore have better established levels for its population than one with a small throughput. This in turn produces more accurate risk estimates on all pregnancies, particularly for those women whose levels do not correlate with the expected norm.

However, in Down's syndrome affected pregnancies it is realised that certain markers may be raised or lowered in the maternal blood and this is the basis of screening assessment of levels to see if they vary from the expected.[10] In Down's syndrome affected pregnancies it is well documented that a pattern exists for the majority of affected pregnancies: the AFP, PAPP-A and uE3 would be lower than expected, and the hCG and inhibin-A would be higher than expected. This can be seen in Figure 9.2 where the normal level is shown as 1 MOM. When a change from the expected is noted, any level which is higher or lower than expected would be compared to see if it falls into a Down's syndrome affected pregnancy pattern. The greater the variation away from the normal then the greater

the risk will be in the final interpretation. The expected pattern for Down's syndrome can be seen in Figure 9.2. Though the levels are not accurate, they give an indication of what would be seen in a Down's affected pregnancy.

MULTIPLES OF THE MEDIAN

Most biochemistry results are given out using the term multiple of the median or MOM. Although it is not imperative to understand the concept behind the interpretation of the result, it can be helpful. A median value is a mathematical term for when a number of results are measured, in this instance blood results from pregnant women, plotted on a line and the middle value taken. For example, if 11 blood results are measured the value of each result may vary from 2 iu (international units) to 15 iu. These might read 2, 4, 4, 5, 6, 6, 8, 10, 12, 12, 15. Though the range is quite extensive from 2 to 15, the median value would be the middle figure on the line, which is 6. Therefore it would be said that 6 is the normal value expected, or the median. This is very different from the mean or average when all the values from 2 to 15 would be added together and then divided by the number of values, in this instance 11. This would give a mean of 7.63. It is accepted that using a median value will give a more accurate overall assessment of the normal level than using a mean or average value because it is less likely to be skewed by extreme results. In a laboratory, values for each marker are calculated separately, as they all vary at different gestations. This was shown in Figure 9.1. Gradually over time the laboratory establishes a large data set of values for their population and are able to establish what the expected value is for each day of gestation. From this it can be deduced what the median for a normal pregnancy should be. Since expected levels in a Down's syndrome affected pregnancy are known from previous research, a risk can be calculated on the basis of how closely the level for any individual resembles the pattern found in a Down's syndrome pregnancy.

Transferring this to the meaning of each marker, if we knew that at 16 weeks the level of AFP normally found in a pregnant woman was 30 iu, then a pregnant woman who had a sample analysed and

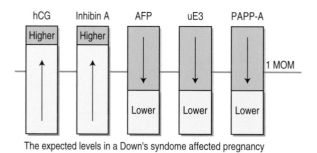

The expected levels in a Down's syndome affected pregnancy

Figure 9.2 Expected levels of biochemical markers in a Down's syndrome affected pregnancy.

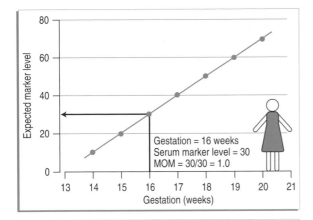

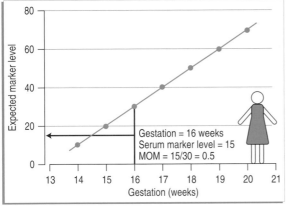

Figure 9.3 MOM values (with kind permission of the National Down's Syndrome Screening Programme, training pack).

had a level of 30 iu would be said to be exactly normal (i.e. the median value for 16 weeks is 30 iu, the woman's level is 30 iu), and this is given as 1 MOM. If she has a level of 60 iu at 16 weeks, this would be twice the value expected and would be given as 2 MOM. If her level was found to be 15 iu, this would be half of what is expected and said to be 0.5 MOM. Figure 9.3 illustrates this.

When discussing the result with a woman and her partner, the levels can be explained in relation to the normal values. However, it should always be stated that it is not known why variation occurs. Some Down's syndrome pregnancies can have normal levels and unaffected pregnancies can often have levels which resemble those of a Down's syndrome pregnancy. These are normal variants but there is no explanation as to why this occurs.

COMBINATION OF MARKERS

The different markers which are used, and which have been described above, can be put together and used in combination to increase the reliability of the test. The combinations commonly used today are the double test, triple test and quadruple test. These are all second trimester tests and give different detection and false-positive rates.

The double test usually consists of AFP and hCG. However, this should no longer be used after April 1st 2005.[11]

The triple test normally consists of AFP, hCG and uE3, and from April 1st 2005 this is the test of choice until further markers are evaluated.

The quadruple test consists of AFP, hCG, uE3 and inhibin-A.

A double test can also be used in the first trimester, consisting of PAPP-A and hCG, but it should always be used in conjunction with nuchal translucency measurement. This is discussed in Chapter 7.

The detection rates for these tests are established by the Health Technology Assessment SURUSS report[8] and set out in the NICE Clinical Guideline.[12]

The variation of markers and the times at which they are used can be very confusing not only for women but for health professionals who are trying to explain this to parents. It is important, therefore, that each local hospital makes its testing strategy clear both for staff and for patients and that these are supported by up to date policies and guidance.

There are also different types of strategies in screening that are now becoming evident. Screening has developed extensively from the use of AFP as the single known marker in 1984 to the variation of tests now possible. Change is ongoing and research is continuing to ensure that the best possible detection and lowest false-positive rates are achieved using the most effective strategies.

Combined screening takes place in the first trimester and this is when hCG, PAPP-A and the nuchal translucency measurement together give an overall risk, usually at 12–13 weeks of pregnancy.

A combination now exists where markers can be added together from the first and second trimester to give an overall detection and false-positive rate. These screening strategies are commonly known as:

- integrated
- serum integrated and (more recently)
- contingency screening.

Integrated screening

The integrated test consists of adding markers such as PAPP-A and a measurement of nuchal translucency in the first trimester then withholding a result until further testing in the second trimester using hCG, uE3, AFP and inhibin-A takes place. These are added together to give an overall result.

Serum integrated screening

The serum integrated test is the same but without the use of the ultrasound screen for nuchal translucency. In both the serum integrated and the integrated screening test, the results of the tests are not disclosed to the woman until the final result is obtained in the second trimester. Some feel that that this two-stage process is not based on sound ethical principles, as information is withheld until the final testing is completed.

Contingency screening

Contingency screening is in its infancy in this country. With this screening strategy any combination of markers can be used but commonly it is hCG PAPP-A and nuchal translucency in the first trimester. This is similar to the integrated testing strategy but the result and the risk are disclosed after the first test and only a proportion of women are offered screening in the second trimester to refine the risk. A cut off value is used, for example 1 in 150 in the first trimester, and if the result is higher than this then a diagnostic procedure is offered at that point. If the result were lower than 1 in 1500 then the woman would not be offered any further screening as it is known that even by performing further tests, the result would never become a high risk. Those women who are given a risk of between 1 in 150 and 1 in 1500 would be offered second trimester screening and a result given based on the combination of first and second trimester markers. As can be realised, this is quite a difficult strategy to implement and for staff to understand until it becomes common practice.

One of the benefits of contingency screening is that women whose risk will not change from a high risk in the first trimester have the option of undergoing a diagnostic test early in the pregnancy rather than waiting until 16 weeks. Conversely, those women whose result is very low in the first trimester of pregnancy would not require any further screening, as it is highly unlikely that their risk, whatever screening tools are used in the second trimester, would change to a higher risk. The proportion of women who would need to be tested in the second trimester is around 10% depending on the various cut off values used.[13]

It is important to remember when offering a screening service that there will always be the need for second trimester screening for those women who present after 14 weeks of pregnancy. This is known to be around 20% of all pregnant women. The policy of the Department of Health is that all women should be offered screening when they present, up until 20 weeks of pregnancy. Therefore it is important that a screening service has in place the ability to offer screening to those women who present later in the pregnancy.

DETECTION RATES AND FALSE-POSITIVE RATES

A detection rate is referred to as a sensitivity rate, and this is more commonly referred to in public health screening programmes. It is the proportion of affected pregnancies detected in the screened population.

The false-positive rate is also known as the specificity rate in public health terminology. This is the number of screening tests who are given a high risk result, but do not have Down's syndrome. Those pregnancies that are given a higher risk and then found to be affected are known as true-positive results. The terminology is explained in more detail in Chapter 2.

As with any screening test, there has to be a cut off value where women are not offered further diagnostic tests to assess the status of the pregnancy. It does not mean that those women will not have an affected pregnancy. It only means that their risk is lower than the cut-off and further diagnostic tests will not be offered. A screening programme is only a risk assessment and there will be certain affected pregnancies that will be missed and not detected. It is important that the woman who presents for screening understands that occasionally an affected pregnancy is not detected. Those women who are given a lower risk result but are subsequently found to have an affected pregnancy are known as false negatives. Those women who are given a lower risk result but have an unaffected pregnancy are known as true negatives.

THE QUALITY OF DOWN'S SYNDROME SCREENING

All of the above screening markers and strategies have different detection and false-positive rates and it is important that local services are able to demonstrate the effectiveness of their own screening programmes.[14]

A population screening programme, such as Down's syndrome screening, should be able to demonstrate that it reaches a certain standard. This is the basis of the Department of Health's policy on best practice.[11] All screening programmes, whatever markers and strategies they use, should be able to reach a detection rate of greater than 75% for a false-positive rate of less than 3% by 2007. It may well be that from 2007 standards will be changed and raised to continually improve the detection rates and lower the false-positive rates of screening programmes to ensure that women get the best possible service. It is now expected that all programmes should be able to demonstrate their effectiveness and standards to women who are using the test and to the public health departments who oversee the safety and quality of population screening programmes.

Safety Issues

The main reason for aiming for a low false-positive rate of less than 3% is to reduce the number of invasive diagnostic techniques that have to be performed. Diagnostic techniques carry with them a risk of miscarriage of the pregnancy and therefore should not be undertaken without careful consideration of the consequences that may occur to the pregnancy. Hopefully, in the future we may be able to lower the false-positive rate to below 3% and

therefore reduce the number of invasive techniques and the number of miscarriages caused by those procedures.[15]

Any screening programme should have a quality assurance aspect incorporated into its process framework and this is no different for Down's syndrome screening. It is vitally important that quality assurance of the screening programme takes place along with facilities to audit and monitor the programme. One of the standards of the UK National Screening Committee is that a programme manager should be accountable and responsible for the quality of the programme, reporting to a clinical governance board any concerns that may arise from the screening pathway.[16] Each hospital should be able to demonstrate that the standard is being reached that and mechanisms are in place to achieve this, including assessment of the quality of the service offered from the point of view of the women who use it.

FACTORS THAT MAY AFFECT THE RISK CALCULATION

There are many different variables and factors which can affect the result of the screening test. When taking the history of a pregnant woman prior to the screening test it is vitally important that these details are passed on to the laboratory so they can include them in the final interpretation of the result. The main factor adversely affecting a screening result is incorrect gestational age of the pregnancy. If the wrong gestation is given then the laboratories will calculate the result incorrectly. This is one of the main reasons for having the age of the pregnancy established by ultrasound dating scan prior to the screening test. Correct gestation of the pregnancy is vital for correct result interpretation.

The level of AFP can be elevated by bleeding in pregnancy. The level of AFP in a Down's affected pregnancy is normally lower than expected. If bleeding has taken place, the AFP level is artificially raised and an incorrect risk is calculated. The risk given will be lower than it actually is. It is therefore prudent to delay taking a screening test until at least 2 weeks after bleeding has stopped. This of course, will not affect first trimester screening and is therefore only a consideration if a second trimester screening programme is in place.

Women who have a larger body mass index generally have lower levels of all biochemical markers. This is because the markers are diluted in larger circulating volumes. It is therefore extremely important when completing information for the laboratory that the weight of the woman is noted on the request form.

It was realised some time ago that women who are diabetics have an effect on the Down's syndrome screening programme. However, this is really only pertinent to those diabetics who are not well controlled. It is now believed that if a diabetic is well controlled then this should have no effect on the interpretation of the levels of the markers. Despite this, it is still important to give full information to the laboratory on the request form.

Multiple pregnancies may cause difficulties in interpreting risks in a biochemical screening programme as the levels are normally twice that expected of a singleton pregnancy. It can be difficult to establish which fetus is affected. The fetus that is normal can influence the levels of the affected fetus and vice versa. In multiple pregnancies the screening test of choice would be nuchal translucency by ultrasound as this will give a more accurate measurement and establish which fetus is affected. It is also known that the smoking status of a pregnant woman markedly affects the levels of inhibin-A. The smoking status of the woman should therefore be identified and noted on the laboratory form. Any level of smoking can alter the inhibin-A measurement by 47%.

Age is a factor taken into account in risk calculation, and in those pregnancies conceived by egg donation it must be remembered that it is the age of the donor which is required, not the age of the woman carrying the fetus. Therefore the woman should be asked for the age of the person who donated the egg and this should be made explicit on the request form.

INTERPRETING THE RISK

Screening for and interpreting biochemical markers for Down's syndrome is a complex issue. The interpretation software used to calculate the risk takes into account a number of parameters and uses a specific algorithm. There are various types of software calculation that can be used but they should all adhere to regulations and standards. All results should be calculated using software which has been specifically designed for Down's syndrome screening. The software used must always have a CE mark measured against European regulations. This came into force in December 2003.

TRISOMY 18

Biochemical screening for trisomy 18 (Edwards syndrome) can take place using the Down's syndrome screening test. The markers used are the same but it is known that the levels differ from a normal or Down's syndrome pregnancy. In a pregnancy affected with Edwards syndrome the levels are all lower than expected. Using its calculation software, the laboratory can give a risk for Edwards syndrome; however, it is possible to detect the majority of cases using a fetal anomaly ultrasound scan, where the abnormal skeletal structures will be seen, and then a diagnostic test to establish the karyotype will be offered.

Key Practice Points

- The risk of having a baby with Down's syndrome is related to maternal age, so screening tests incorporate this background risk with levels of biochemical markers.
- Since biochemical markers vary with gestational age, accurate dating scans are required for calculation of risk results.
- Detection rates and false-positive rates improve when appropriate biochemical markers are combined.
- Low false-positive rates improve the safety of Down's syndrome screening because fewer diagnostic tests will mean fewer procedure-induced miscarriages.
- Bleeding in pregnancy can increase AFP levels and falsely lower the Down's syndrome risk result.
- Weight should be recorded on request forms, as increased body mass index and circulating blood volume dilutes the levels of biochemical markers.
- Biochemical screening is not reliable for multiple pregnancies.
- The age of the donor should be recorded for pregnancies conceived through egg donation.

References

1. Langdon Down J. Observations on an ethnic classification of idiots. Clinical Lectures and Reports, London Hospital 1864; 3:259–262.

2. Steel MW, Breg WR. Chromosome analysis of human amniotic fluid cells. Lancet 1966 (Feb 19); 1(7434):383–385.

3. Cuckle HS, Wald NJ, Lindenbaum RH. Maternal serum alpha–feto protein measurement. A screening test for Down's syndrome. Lancet 1984; 323(8383):926–929.

4. Bogart M, Pandian MR, Jones OW. Abnormal maternal serum chorionic gonadotrophin levels in pregnancies with fetal chromosomal abnormalilties. Prenata Diagnosis 1987 (Nov); 7:623–630.

5. Snijders RJM, Noble P, Sebire N, et al. UK multicentre project on assessment of risk of trisomy 21 by maternal age and fetal nuchal-translucency thickness at 10–14 weeks of gestation. Lancet 1998; 352 (9125):343–346.

6. Cuckle HS, Wald NJ, Thompson SG. Estimating a woman's risk of having a pregnancy associated with Down's syndrome using her age and serum alphafetoprotein level. British Journal of Obstetrics and Gynaecology 1987 (May); 94(5):387–402.

7. Cuckle HS, Aitken D, Goodburn S, et al. Age standardisation when target setting and auditing performance of Down syndrome screening programmes. Prenatal Diagnosis 2004 (Nov); 24(11):851–856.

8. Wald NJ, Rodeck C, Hackshaw AK, et al. First and second trimester antenatal screening for Down's syndrome: the results of the Serum, Urine and Ultrasound Screening Study (SURUSS). Health Technol Assess 2003; 7(11):1–77.

9. Rudnicka AR, Wald NJ, Huttly W, Hackshaw AK. Influence of maternal smoking on the birth prevalence of Down's syndrome and on second trimester screening performance. Prenatal Diagnosis 2002 (Oct); 22(10):893–897.

10. Wald NJ, Kennard A, Densem J, et al. Antenatal maternal serum screening for Down's syndrome: results of a demonstration project. BMJ 1992; 305(6850):391–394.

11. Department of Health. Model of best practice. Down's syndrome screening. London: Department of Health; November 2003.

12. Royal College of Obstetricians and Gynaecologists, National Institute for Clinical Excellence. Antenatal care: routine care for the healthy pregnant woman. Clinical Guideline. London: RCOG, NICE; 2003.

13. Wright D, Bradbury I, Benn P, et al. Contingent screening for Down's syndrome is an efficient alternative to non-disclosure sequential screening. Prenat Diagn 2004 (Oct); 24(10):762–766.

14. Wellesley D, Boyle T, Barber J, Howe D. Retrospective audit of different antenatal screening policies for Down's syndrome in eight district general hospitals in one health region. BMJ 2002 (July); 325(7354):15.

15. The Canadian Early and Mid-Trimester Amniocentesis Trial (CEMAT) Group. Randomised trial to assess safety and fetal outcome of early and midtrimester amniocentesis. Lancet 1998; 351: (9098):242–247.

16. UK National Screening Committee. Antenatal screening standards incorporating standards for Down's syndrome screening. Oxford: UK National Screening Committee, Institute of Health Sciences; 2004.

10

Chromosomal and genetic testing

Danna Kirwan

INTRODUCTION

The discovery of pregnancy complications evokes a considerable degree of anxiety and distress for the majority of women. Medicalised care or hospitalisation may prevent the privilege of pregnancy choice. In essence, there is a danger that the 'condition' not the woman becomes the central focus. Thus, if pregnancy is perceived as illness, then women are treated as patients. As a consequence, the once positive woman may manifest feelings of dependency, isolation, boredom, stress, frustration, loss of identity, and feelings of worthlessness, powerlessness and negativity, recognised by several authors who describe how 'high-risk' pregnancies change one's perspective of life.[1-5]

The use of technology, such as ultrasound, and invasive procedures for the diagnosis of genetic and chromosomal disorders has indeed 'medicalised' pregnancy and redefined its position within maternity services in a way that could be likened to a 'pendulum shift'.[6] Technology brings with it many wonderful interventions to 'make it all better', but unfortunately the intrusion can give rise to anxiety and fear, especially where the procedure involves invading the pregnancy.

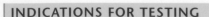

INDICATIONS FOR TESTING

For the majority of women, pregnancy is a normal life event, one considered to be a happy and momentous occasion. There are a variety of experiences during pregnancy which influence how women feel and behave. Some women will remember the event for the rest of their lives, particularly when it is a problematic experience.

Indications for prenatal diagnosis can be divided broadly into five groups:

- Abnormal maternal serum biochemistry either in the first or second trimester of pregnancy, such as found through integrated, combined, serum integrated, triple or quadruple test. This is discussed in more detail in Chapter 9.
- Maternal anxiety request.
- A previous history of either a structural, chromosomal or genetic abnormality such as trisomy 13, 18 or 21.
- A familial genetic history of a disorder such as cystic fibrosis, Duchenne muscular dystrophy, Tay-Sachs disease, sickle cell disease or thalassaemia.
- Abnormal findings on ultrasound scan, either in the first or second trimester of pregnancy, such as a neural tube defect, gross cystic hygroma, exomphalos or gastroshisis.

Antenatal care, advocated by midwives to monitor and promote wellbeing in pregnancy, can be likened to a Pandora's box.[7] On the surface, it provides care and support. Within this package is offered reassurance, which undoubtedly sounds attractive to women, but can escalate into an array of problems if not fully understood. Unfortunately, the concepts of prenatal screening are not well understood either by healthcare professionals or pregnant women. Thus, the offer of what appears to be a simple blood test or ultrasound scan can spiral into an emotional roller coaster of ethical dilemmas and emotional events. For instance, a positive test result for Down's syndrome screening suddenly transforms what was once considered a 'normal' pregnancy into a high-risk context. Similarly, the discovery of a variance from the 'normal' on a routine first or second pregnancy scan requires further investigation to either confirm or refute a structural fetal abnormality. In contrast, having previously had a child with a problem, or having a family history of a condition can heighten awareness of the worst possible case scenario, resulting in considerable anxiety.

USE OF INVASIVE PROCEDURES

The utilisation of ultrasound in pregnancy, since its introduction in the mid 1950s, has revolutionised the field of medicine. The specialty of fetal medicine was born. In addition to the use of ultrasound for the surveillance of fetal defects, the use of a variety of invasive tests meant that suspicious findings *in utero* could either be confirmed or refuted by using fetal tissue samples. It is not uncommon to find that some individuals perceive prenatal diagnosis as a precursor to termination of pregnancy, since this choice is sometimes made. Much depends on the nature of the problem that is found. However, prenatal diagnosis can also be considered as a proactive measure in that healthcare professionals, on discovering a problem, can actively plan and engage the parents in the management and treatment of the baby's condition in utero or after the birth.

PREREQUISITES FOR INVASIVE TESTING

This section of this chapter focuses on the prerequisites for invasive testing, in particular pre-test communication, as a preparation for invasive testing, and how this is delivered within the clinical setting.

Pre-test discussions

A prerequisite of any invasive procedure is to ensure that women and their partners are fully prepared about the process of testing. It is essential that a good rapport is established with the woman, as this will encourage trust and hopefully reduce anxiety. The facilitation of informed decisions is a vital part of any procedure carried out in medicine, particularly where problems exist. This requires a supporting and nurturing approach, where the carer provides an arena to enable a woman or a couple to reach a decision that they are comfortable with. It is paramount that the woman is given time to make an 'informed decision'. This means being given time to digest what she has been told, and the opportunity to reflect and ask questions and, if necessary, come back another day with a decision. This is discussed in more detail in Chapter 2. An environment conducive to privacy and calm should be provided, one which guarantees no interruptions. After all there is much to consider and contemplate which may affect the woman's life thereafter. The provision of written as well as verbal information about the procedure is important, so special provision should be made for those individuals for whom English is not a first language. Other portals of information may be useful in aiding understanding such as video, CD-ROM, audio-cassette or DVD. Ethical and moral beliefs should also be taken into consideration. Not all hospital trusts adopt the practice of formal written consent. However, the conversation about the procedure should be clearly documented in the practitioner's hospital or hand-held case notes.

Evidence suggests that psychological support and comfort for the pregnant woman during a stressful procedure minimises pain and anxiety.[8] At times of stress, people forget quite a large proportion of the information that is given to them verbally. There is a need, therefore, to reinforce verbal information in other ways, either through the provision of accessible printed or recorded information or through the provision of support services within the hospital after consultation.[9]

Good communication

All healthcare professionals involved in pregnancy care require communication and interpersonal skills. These are essential to their role. In particular, highly developed skills are important when caring for women with complicated pregnancies in order to ensure that they truly understand what they are experiencing. It is essential that they do not feel inadequately informed about their progress and treatment. The extent to which professionals are able to use these skills directly affects a woman's experience of care and may have implications for her pregnancy as a whole.[10]

It cannot be assumed that all people are the same. Different levels of communication are neces-

sary for different individuals, much depending on their existing knowledge and ability to understand. Healthcare professionals need to be aware of these issues and be able to adapt to appropriately. The importance of an inclusive partnership has also been recognised, where the 'balance of power' is shared between parents and carers.

The healthcare professional involved in the discussion should be knowledgeable, confident and competent to provide information about the practical aspects and implications of the procedure. This should be carried out in an unhurried manner, particularly as invasive testing is related to fetal loss. Box 10.1 lists the topics that midwives, doctors or other professionals involved in counselling women for prenatal diagnosis should ideally cover during their discussions.

PERFORMING THE TESTS

Ultrasound underpins fetal invasive testing and the operator who will be performing the test should always carry out a detailed ultrasound scan to attain information about the gestational age and viability of the fetus, the number of fetuses and the presence of any apparent anomalies. The location of the fetus in relation to adjacent structures should also be noted, along with the following:

- Placental position
- Amount of liquor present
- Optimal amniotic pool for retrieving an amniotic fluid sample

---

Box 10.1 Topics to be covered in pre-test discussions

- Aims of invasive testing
- Indications for testing
- Nature of the procedure
- Accuracy of results
- Complications of testing—laboratory, fetal and maternal
- Limitations of the test
- Length of time to results and method of reporting
- Methods of termination for abnormal results.

- Tissue depth (from skin to target pool) as the latter will aid the operator in selecting an appropriate needle size that is sufficient in length to reach the amniotic pool (or placenta for the purposes of chorionic villus sampling (CVS)).

Findings from this baseline scan can provide further information on whether to continue with invasive testing. For example, finding a lethal congenital anomaly may influence the woman to decline invasive testing. Similarly, evidence of bleeding may defer the procedure until such time when the bleeding stops.

Operator skills

The Royal College of Obstetricians and Gynaecologists (RCOG) stipulates that any 'practitioner carrying out ultrasound as a part of the amniocentesis or CVS procedure should be trained to the competencies of RCOG/RCR Diploma in Obstetric Ultrasound level or equivalent'.[11] The college believes that experienced operators, who maintain their expertise by working within a fetal medicine environment, should supervise training. This ensures a high throughput of anomaly scans and needling procedures. Additionally, the guideline recommends that: 'Competence is best assessed through continuous audit of complications such as "need for second insertion" and "miscarriage rate".'[11] The past few years have also witnessed the development of midwives such as myself performing ultrasound and invasive testing.[12] It is recognised that midwives working in fetal medicine specialties are in an ideal position to provide counselling and intervention for high-risk pregnancy.[13,14]

Environment and organisation of care

The organisation of care should include high specification equipment, a robust framework for training, and links with related services such as cytogenetic and molecular genetics laboratories and medical genetic services. Facilities for carrying out pregnancy termination and follow-up clinical counselling and support are also essential. Overall, ultrasound and testing should be carried out within a calm and quiet environment, conducive to concentrating and working in a coordinated manner. Staff should try and minimise the clinical aspect of the area, by creating a 'home from home' environment so as to promote comfort and ease distress. Anything other than this would evoke additional unnecessary stress. In many centres, staff aim to dress informally rather than wear uniform, but this is a matter for debate in relation to infection control policies in some Trusts.

Preparation

It is customary for another individual such as the woman's partner, other family member or friend to accompany and support the woman during the procedure. It is always wise to check before the procedure begins that the woman does not have a needle phobia. It is essential that once on the examination couch the woman is made comfortable, and that a pillow or small latex wedge is placed under her back so as to avoid supine hypotension, particularly if the procedure is carried out within the third trimester of pregnancy.

The garments covering the abdominal area should be moved in order to expose the area. Dignity and privacy should be maintained by placing a cotton sheet or paper drape below the lower abdomen and over the legs. It must never be assumed that the ultrasound monitor should be turned towards the woman as according to Garrett and Charlton[15] some women would prefer not to see the baby during the procedure, especially if the pregnancy was unplanned, as this may add to feelings of guilt.

Despite invasive testing being considered as relatively simple, precautions should always be taken to minimise the risk of infection to both the woman and fetus. It is necessary to thoroughly clean the abdominal area with an antiseptic product. Policy varies amongst operators, but the most commonly used agents are sterile alcohol (Alcowipes) or 2.5 % chlorhexidine gluconate solution.

Obviously, women wish to minimise discomfort or pain during a needling procedure. For this reason 'numbing' the abdominal skin and uterine peritoneum is an option. However, the injection of 1 ml of 0.5 % lidocaine can be more of an uncomfortable experience than the original procedure and women should be informed of this. Amniocentesis is generally relatively quick and simple to perform and the needle has a very fine gauge. Local anaesthetic may be more appropriate for CVS, as the sampling needles are slighter longer and wider to allow tissue to pass within the needle shaft. Overall, this procedure takes a little longer.

TECHNIQUES USED FOR DIAGNOSTIC TESTING

The three main invasive tests, namely amniocentesis, CVS and cordocentesis, are all performed as outpatient procedures. These are described with particular emphasis on the indications for the tests. The risks and benefits are also explained.

Amniocentesis

According to the RCOG, amniocentesis is the most common invasive prenatal diagnostic procedure undertaken in the UK. It is the transabdominal surgical removal of amniotic fluid under direct ultrasound guidance for a variety of purposes, primarily for the diagnosis of chromosomal and genetic disorders.

The technique has a long history. It was first developed in Germany in the 1880s to decompress polyhydramnios[16,17] and then utilised in the 1930s by Menees et al to inject contrast media to visualise the fetus and placenta.[18] In 1937 Aburel used the technique for performing in utero termination of pregnancy[19] by injecting hypertonic saline into the amniotic fluid and in the mid 1950s Bevis and Walker developed the procedure of aspirating liquor at 2-weekly intervals to quantify the amount of haemoglobin breakdown, otherwise known as erythroblastosis, for women affected by rhesus disease.[20,21]

It was not until 1956 when fetal sexing was discovered, that the brave new world of chromosomal and genetic analysis begain.[22] Steele and Breg followed by demonstrating and reporting that cultured cells were indeed suitable for analysing the number and type of chromosomes of the unborn child.[23] Two years later, the first chromosomal abnormality, Down's syndrome, was detected.[24,25] The range of uses for amniotic fluid continued to grow, and in 1972 Brock and Sutcliffe discovered that an excess amount of alpha-fetoprotein (AFP) was associated with neural tube defects.[26]

Timing of the procedure

Amniocentesis can be carried out from as early as 15 weeks' gestation up to full term. The timing of amniocentesis is generally dependent on the reason for referral. However, most operators carry out the procedure for fetal karyotype purposes following antenatal serum screening for Down's syndrome at around 15–20 weeks' gestation. At this gestation, the amount of amniotic fluid is around 150–200 ml. Both the RCOG and UK National Screening Committee (NSC) recommend that the procedure be performed no earlier than 15 weeks' gestation, as before this the fusion between chorionic and amniotic membranes is incomplete and this could potentially encourage a rupture of the membranes. Furthermore, fetal loss rates are known to be higher before 15 weeks and there is a 'ten fold increase in the incidence of fetal talipes'.[28,11,12,27,29]

Early amniocentesis (less than 15 weeks' gestation) is known to be associated with other additional complications, such as insufficient and immature amniocytes, or ruptured membranes that can inadvertently cause oligohydramnios or anhydramnnios. This can result in miscarriage or pulmonary hypoplasia, leading to severe respiratory problems in the newborn period.

Ultrasound prior to the procedure

As previously mentioned, the procedure should always be carried out using 'real time' ultrasound equipment, under continuous ultrasound control. This minimises the risk of injury to the fetus and the woman as there is continuous monitoring of the needle throughout its entry in the womb and, as a consequence, the rates of 'blood taps' are lowered.[30,33] Most doctors or midwives performing the procedure tend to use a linear or curvilinear ultrasound probe, as this ensures that they can clearly visualise the point of entry (skin) to the pool of amniotic fluid.

Surgical technique

Some operators, like myself, perform amniocentesis single handedly, whilst others have an assistant to aspirate the fluid. It is essential to produce the best ultrasound image quality so that the needle can be safely guided through the various tissue layers as listed in Box 10.2. The whole length of the needle should be observed during the process so as to ensure proper needle placement. Thus, the practice of 'blind' needling, which involves palpating the outline of the uterus and inserting a needle into a selected pool without ultrasound, is not recommended as injury may occur to either the fetus or the maternal organs (bowel, bladder or reproductive organs).

Having performed an ultrasound scan and positioned the woman in a supine position, the operator would begin the procedure by cleansing and numbing the abdominal skin. The stylet of the needle is removed and with a 20 ml syringe attached on the hub of the needle, gentle suction should be applied to withdraw a few millilitres of fluid as vigorous traction could draw on the membranes and cause shearing. If blood-stained initially, the first few millilitres are discarded and a clean syringe is attached. With the syringe attached again, suction is applied to continue the process until 20 ml of fluid are aspirated. The fluid is then put into a sterile bottle, labelled with the woman's hospital casenote number, full name, date of birth and demographic details. During the procedure, the operator and midwifery staff should reassure the woman to reduce her anxiety.

Planning and precision of needling have to be carefully executed, as the aim is to obtain a sample at the first attempt. As I discovered, performing amniocentesis presents new challenges each time, simply because not all pregnancies behave in the same way. Some fetuses are very active and mobile within the womb; placental positions can vary, which will result in the operator having to change tactics. Overall, common sense, intuition and vigilance are required to 'tap' the sac successfully. Sometimes a full bladder is advantageous, whilst on other occasions it may make the procedure more difficult to perform.

Ideally, the operator should avoid the placenta when inserting the needle; however, where a clear 'window' is not present, then passing the needle through the placenta is acceptable. However, the operator should be cautious and avoid going into the placental edge, umbilical cord or cord insertion. Most operators use a 22 gauge, 9 cm needle for aspiration, as shown in Figure 10.1. Overall, women describe the experience as being uncomfortable and similar to having venepuncture. However, slight pain can be experienced when the needle enters the uterine peritoneum.

Needling problems

Occasionally, problems during the procedure can occur which in experienced hands can be quickly resolved. After inserting the needle into the amniotic pool, if after suction no fluid is retrieved, this could be due to needle blockage by 'debris' (maternal tissue) or incomplete piercing of the two membranes. Rotating the needle within the skin can relieve the problem, but if after applying suction again fluid still does not come up into the syringe, then reinserting the stylet and gently

---

Box 10.2 Amniocentesis—the anatomical tissue layers the needle passes through during procedure

- Skin
- Fat
- Abdominal muscle
- Uterine peritoneum
- Uterus
- Thinnest edge of placenta (where placenta is within target area)
- Chorion and amnion membranes
- Pool of liquor.

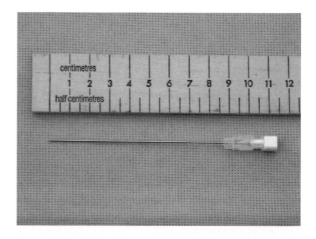

Figure 10.1 Amniocentesis needle (20g × 9 cm).

pushing the needle in a little further should rectify the problem.

Figure 10.2 shows a sample of amniotic fluid. Amniotic fluid or liquor is a versatile medium, straw coloured in appearance, very similar to urine. It basically comprises fetal urine, desquamated cells from the fetal skin, gastrointestinal tract, genitourinary and respiratory tracts, and amnion.[34] 'Bloody taps' or a blood-stained sample should be taken seriously, as this could be a result of fetal or maternal injury or previous intra-amniotic bleeding. The fetal heart should be checked, particularly where there is fresh blood. If the bleeding is fresh, the procedure should be abandoned and the woman brought back for monitoring. If the sample is blood-stained, this could be due to the puncturing of the uterus or a previous intra-amniotic bleed. Cytogenetic laboratories prefer a clear sample as a blood-stained sample can interfere with analysis, particularly if rapid result technologies are to be employed (see later). The RCOG stipulates that no more than two needle attempts should be made and where any difficulties arise the advice of a senior colleague who is experienced in the procedure should be sought.[11]

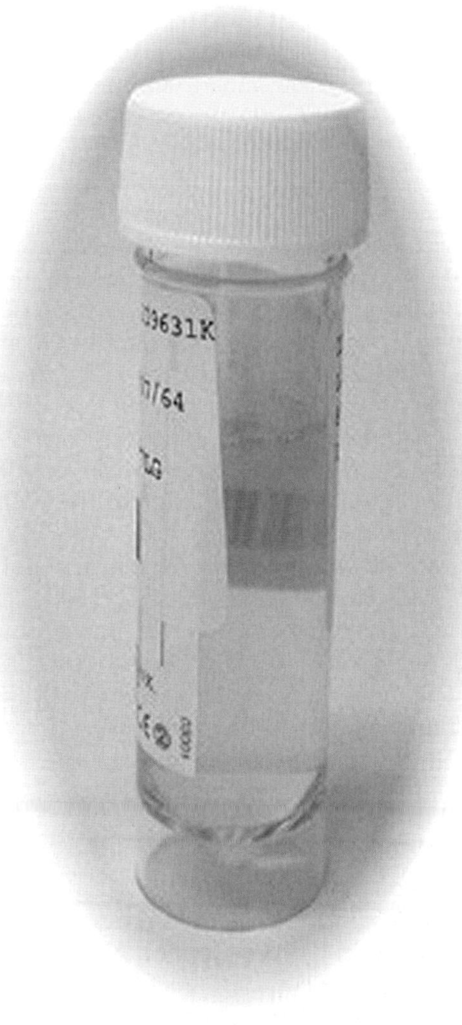

Chorionic villus sampling (CVS)

The introduction of first trimester invasive testing made it possible to detect chromosomal and genetic disorders much earlier in pregnancy. The procedure of CVS was introduced in the mid 1980s. It meant that women who choose to end their pregnancy do not have to endure the feeling of fetal movement prior to mid-trimester termination of pregnancy. Hence, some individuals find the test more acceptable than amniocentesis. The procedure of CVS, also known as chorionic villus biopsy, tends to be performed for the following reasons:

- Advanced maternal age
- A history of a previous affected child
- A family history of genetic disease, particularly where there is a history of an autsomal recessive disorder (mother and father are carriers of the disorder) e.g. Tay-Sachs, haemoglobinopathy, cystic fibrosis
- A familial history of an autsomal dominant disorder such as Duchenne muscular dystrophy.

The procedure involves taking a sample of the chorion frondosum via transabdominal or transcervical routes. Small samples of chorionic villi are removed under continuous ultrasound guidance. The chorion frondosum, the early developing placenta, is a microscopic, soft, thickened area of villi (projections), which by 9 weeks' gestation is approximately 1.0–1.5 cm thick. The cells that make up the chorionic villi are of fetal origin.

The procedure was first developed by Mohr in Scandinavia[35] then adopted by the Far East for determining fetal sex for sex-selection.[36] However,

Figure 10.2 Amniocentesis sample for laboratory analysis. The colour of the sample has the appearance of white wine.

it was only in the early 1980s that it came to be used with ultrasound guidance.[34]

In its infancy, the procedure was carried out from before 10 weeks' gestation. However, due to the findings reporting incidences of prenatal abnormality, it became the subject of public interest when Firth and colleagues in Oxford reported a cluster of five babies with congenital limb and facial reduction defects, otherwise known as oromandibular limb hypoplasia, out of 289 pregnancies that underwent CVS.[37] Similarly, other doctors experienced the same phenomenon.[38–40] As result of this, a concerted European action stipulated that the timeframe for CVS be moved up to 10 weeks. So why does this happen? Liu[41] assumes that the cause of the abnormalities is basically biological. Needling the early developing placenta causes subchorionic disruption, which in turn causes uterine contractions. As a consequence, this leads to vasospasm and hypoperfusion in the placenta, which results in the distal fetal limbs and face being starved of blood and nutrients, resulting in absent or short limb buds, micrognathia, microglossia and facial clefting.[41]

Rodeck[42] felt that CVS offered several advantages over amniocentesis:

- The sample obtained is fetal tissue and is therefore genetically and chromosomally identical to the fetus.
- It is accessible during the first trimester by a natural passage, i.e. the cervical canal.
- It can be obtained without perforation of the membranes around the fetus.
- The parents may benefit because there is less delay, termination of pregnancy if indicated is simple, and the physical and psychological traumas of second trimester termination are avoided.

Green[43] also felt that CVS was less stressful for women than amniocentesis (see Box 10.3).

CVS is certainly advantageous in that it provides an early means of obtaining a fetal karyotype or genotype. However, women should be informed that CVS results are difficult to interpret in approximately 1% of cases, since abnormal cell lines can be present in the placenta and not in the fetus. Sometimes, normal and abnormal cell lines may be present in the same placenta. The phenomenon whereby placental cell lines differ from fetal cell lines is known as confined placental mosaicism

---

Box 10.3   Reasons why women choose to have chorionic villus sampling

- They do not have to wait so long to have the test done (10 weeks after their last period instead of 16)
- They do not have to wait so long for results (1 week versus 3 or 4)
- Termination of pregnancy, if indicated can be carried out in the first trimester and thus by dilatation and curettage rather than by inducing labour at 20 weeks or more.

(CPM). When this is suspected, women are offered an amniocentesis for confirmation, as amniocytes are derived from the fetus itself and not the placenta. Experienced cytogenetic laboratories and fetal medicine subspecialists ensure that CPM results are interpreted appropriately, so that inappropriate clinical decisions are avoided.

As with amniocentesis, CVS is offered as an outpatient appointment. Placental localisation determines whether the operator performs the procedure through the vagina and cervix (transcervically) or through the abdomen (transabdominally). Again, CVS must always be performed by an individual who regularly performs the procedure and is confident and competent to do so under continuous ultrasound guidance. Thus, it is usually performed in fetal medicine centres.[11]

Ultrasound imagery in the first trimester of pregnancy does not produce relatively good images because the volume of amniotic fluid during this time is very small (usually around 200–400 ml). Thus, for the purposes of CVS, women are asked to drink fluids and maintain a full bladder.

Transabdominal CVS

This route is used when the placental site is located on the anterior or lateral surface of the uterus. The skin preparation for the procedure is exactly the same as for amniocentesis. However, because CVS tends to be a slightly longer procedure than amniocentesis, doctors tend to offer women local anaesthesia to numb the skin as previously described. A range of specially designed needles can be used for biopsy purposes. Figure 10.3 shows an example of one model commonly used

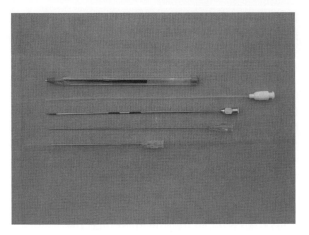

Figure 10.3 Transabdominal chorion sampling needle, third needle up from the bottom (18g × 10 cm). Note that it is slightly thicker and longer than an amniocentesis needle.

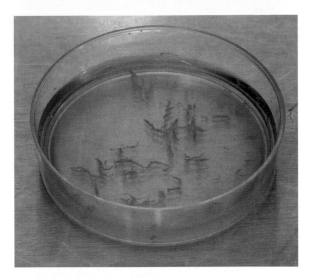

Figure 10.4 Petri dish containing chorion floating in culture medium.

in fetal medicine centres. It comprises a 20-gauge trocar within an 18-gauge needle. The needle is inserted through the abdominal wall, through the peritoneum and into the chorionic plate where the villi are present. Gently moving the needle forwards and backwards within the skin disrupts some villi and the sample is obtained by applying suction with either a syringe or an electrical suction device, otherwise known as 'hoovering'. An alternative method is putting small biopsy forceps down the length of the needle to biopsy a sample. Once the sample is retrieved it is placed in a culture medium to prevent the tissue from dehydrating (see Fig. 10.4).

Transcervical CVS

As mentioned, this method is usually performed if the placenta is posterior to the abdominal wall and requires the woman to adopt a lithotomy position. After thoroughly cleansing the genital and vaginal area with an antiseptic solution, a sterile speculum is inserted into the vagina, the speculum opened, and the cervix also cleansed. With a sonographer scanning the pregnancy, the operator inserts either a catheter or biopsy forceps as shown in Figure 10.5 through the cervix and into the uterus whilst simultaneously watching its passage on the ultrasound monitor. Similarly to the transabdominal method, 'hoovering' is used to retrieve the villi.

Cordocentesis

The removal of blood for the purposes of laboratory analysis, known as cordocentesis (percutaneous umbilical cord blood sampling (PUBS), fetal blood sampling or funipuncture), was first described in 1983.[44] Freda and Adamson[45] first described gaining access to the fetal circulation for the purpose of exchange transfusion via hysterotomy, and in utero cord blood sampling using fibreoptics and fetoscopy followed in the late 1970s.[46]

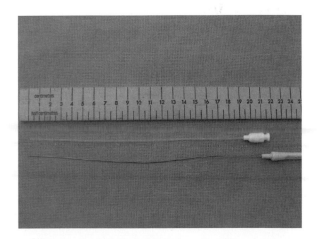

Figure 10.5 Transcervical chorion sampling catheter (below) and trocar. The trocar is made of aluminum and guides the catheter through the cervix.

The three vessels within the umbilical cord are extremely small, particularly so before 18 weeks' gestation. Thus, cordocentesis is an intricate procedure, which requires a great deal of skill, patience and precision. There are several sites for obtaining blood as shown in Box 10.4.

Most operators obtain blood by entering the intrahepatic portal vein or placental cord insertion, as there is minimal risk of haemorrhage.[44] However, if this method or others described prove technically difficult, then direct cardiac puncture can be used as a last resort.[47]

Until recently, results from this method had a turnaround time of around 24–48 hours from sampling. However, with the advancement of molecular genetic technology, cells obtained from amniocentesis and CVS can be analysed in similar timescales. This will be explained in more detail below. A full discussion around the tests available should take place in order for the woman and her partner to understand the risks, benefits and consequences of the procedure and make a truly informed decision.

Fetal blood as a medium for analysis has many benefits, as a wide variety of tests can be per-

Box 10.4 Sites for cordocentesis

- Umbilical vein at the placental cord insertion
- Intrahepatic umbilical vein
- Free loop of cord
- Cardiac chamber

formed. These depend on the indication for sampling and are shown in Table 10.1.

As the method of testing becomes more complex, the risk of pregnancy loss increases. Cordocentesis in particular, compared to the previous methods mentioned, is a more risky procedure. Entering the fetal circulation can potentially induce bradycardia, dysrythmia, haemorrhage or infection. Additionally, a fetus that is already in a compromised state of health due to intrauterine growth retardation (IUGR), chromosomal or genetic anomaly, or hydrops as a consequence of rhesus disease or viral illness, is far more susceptible to complications than a pregnancy deemed high risk following Down's syndrome screening.

The need to enter the fetal circulation, however, in some instances cannot be avoided. This emergency measure could be fruitful in restoring fetal wellbeing. For example, a pregnancy affected by rhesus disease may require an intravascular fetal transfusion of packed red cells to restore a low fetal haemoglobin. This procedure, at or before 20 weeks' gestation, carries a 10–20% risk of fetal mortality.[48]

The therapeutic use of cordocentesis does not end there, as using the cord for the infusion of a variety of drugs can successfully treat other conditions. Similar to the infusion of packed red cells for rhesus disease, platelets can be given to treat thrombocytopenia and anti-arrythmic drugs to correct tachyarrythmia. Additionally, operators may also use this portal as a means for anaesthesia, by giving agents to both sedate and immobilise the

Table 10.1 Clinical indications and investigations for cytogenetic and molecular genetic investigations

Indication	Example	Test	Laboratory
Antenatal serum screening Inherited blood disorders	Raised risk result > 1:250 Haemoglobinopathies Duchenne muscular dystrophy	Karyotyping DNA studies	Cytogenetics Molecular genetics
Suspected fetal infection	Toxoplasmosis Parvovirus	TORCH screen	Virology Bacteriology
Rhesus iso-immunisation IUGR	Red cell antibodies	Spectrophotometry Blood gases/acid–base balance	Chemical pathology Haematology
Neonatal alloimmune thrombocytopenia (NAIT)	Low fetal platelet count	Full blood count	Haematology

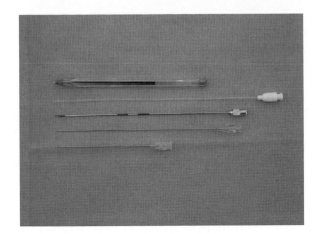

Figure 10.6 Cordocentesis needle for fetal blood sampling (20g × 15 cm), second needle up from the bottom.

fetus in order to carry out feticide or fetal reduction for multiple pregnancy.

Most operators use a 6-inch 22-gauge, needle for cordocentesis. This is shown in Figure 10.6, alongside other sampling needles. Note in Figure 10.7 the difference in appearance and size to the other sampling needles. Also the relative size of the tips in comparison to the head of a matchstick. The cordocentesis needle has a bevelled edge (echo-tip), which makes it easier to see on ultrasound. As the mid-trimester fetus lies within a deep pool of amniotic fluid, a longer needle is required to enable the operator get

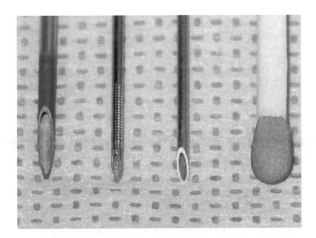

Figure 10.7 Three sampling needles for prenatal diagnosis. Note the difference in appearance and size of the needle tips compared to a matchstick. The cordocentesis needle (middle) has a bevelled edge, specifically designed so that it can be easily seen on ultrasound.

access to the umbilical cord and the small gauge allows just a very tiny hole to be created within the delicate cord vessel, which can go into vasospasm.

Having the inside of the needle coated with silicone reduces the chance of clotting, either during sampling or during intravascular transfusion of blood or platelets. Usually operators target the placental cord insertion or 'free' loop of cord. However, the latter can prove difficult, particularly if the fetus is very mobile.

Once the needle is inserted into the cord vein, the stylet of the needle is removed and gentle suction is applied using small syringes to remove fetal blood for analysis. There is continuous monitoring of the fetal heartbeat with ultrasound. Depending on the tests required, varying amounts of fetal blood are taken for analysis. From 18 weeks of pregnancy, 2–4 ml of blood can be taken without compromising fetal health. Following cordocentesis, it is not uncommon for women to experience a decrease in fetal movement, particularly when the fetus has received sedation. It can be several hours before a fetus resumes activity. It is paramount that women are informed of this and given reassurance before going home.

CARE AFTER PRENATAL DIAGNOSIS

Several healthcare professionals have recognised the need for supporting women and their partners during prenatal diagnosis as a major contribution to antenatal care.[6,12,13,14] Following invasive testing women, although they may be relieved, tend to still feel anxious, weary and sometimes tearful, and thus welcome the offer of sitting or lying down for a short period before going home. Ideally, women and their partners should be placed in a private quiet area, where they can relax and take their time to get themselves together. Midwives should always be prepared for such eventualities and should ensure that women and their partners have the opportunity to ask any questions about the procedure that may be concerning them.

The physical and physiological needs of women also need consideration and this is particularly relevant to advising on possible symptoms to expect after the test; it is also important to ensure that women who are Rhesus D negative are offered antenatal anti-D prophylaxis, as stipulated by recent government health policies.[49–51]

As a matter of good practice, the counselling and giving of information to women and their partners should be documented within hospital and maternal casenotes, and written information should be available to be taken home for private reading as most of the information provided at this time may be forgotten. The discussion should also include the process of how the woman and her partner will receive the test results from the diagnostic procedure. The way in which test results are given may vary amongst hospital trusts, depending on unit policy. Thus, the midwife should obtain telephone numbers and have some idea about the woman's lifestyle so that communication can be made at an appropriate time, fitting in with the woman's routine. Some women work during the day and are only available in the evening, while others do not work, but may prefer a phone call in the evening so their partner can be with them should the result be abnormal. Women should also be made aware of the fact that they may experience abdominal tenderness for a few days following the procedure. They should know how to contact professionals in the event of vaginal bleeding, significant abdominal pain, fever or suspected rupture of membranes. The average time between a procedure and a related pregnancy loss is 3 weeks, although women may experience bleeding or pain before that time.

Overall, it is important for midwives to ensure that whatever the outcome, mutual trust is created through regular communication with the woman and her partner. This is a time of great anxiety and should a test result be abnormal, then the woman will need the support of healthcare professionals. In particular, where a result is abnormal, it is paramount that the woman is informed quickly as she will need time to contemplate a decision about her pregnancy. All Trusts should have in place policies advising midwives of the processes that ensure a swift medical referral for counselling purposes. The small number of women who learn that their baby is affected by a disorder have three options, and it is entirely up to them to choose the one that is best for them. Some will decide to continue the pregnancy and prepare themselves for the challenges they might face bringing up their child. Others may feel unable to bring up a child with a disorder and decide upon adoption. Others may prefer to end their pregnancy. In the time spent in discussion after the procedure the midwife should reassure the woman that whatever her decision, it will be supported.

COMPLICATIONS OF PRENATAL DIAGNOSIS

Without doubt, though testing for birth defects may be routine, it raises a number of troubling issues, especially around the potential for fetal or maternal complications. Although operators may be competent and confident practitioners, even in experienced hands unexpected things may follow. Table 10.2 provides a list of problems that can occur.

It is not uncommon for women undergoing these tests to experience discomfort or pain. The very fact that a needle has pierced the uterus can induce a wave of small contractions, which may require the woman to take oral analgesia. Obviously, experiencing pain can cause anxiety as it may be assumed that miscarriage is occurring and women should be forewarned to expect some discomfort for a day or two afterwards. The midwife should advise the woman, where possible to avoid activities that involve any manual work, lifting, bending or stretching. Although there is no evidence that avoiding physical activity prevents miscarriage, avoiding these tasks appears to be psychologically comforting to women as taking rest makes them feel that they are helping the pregnancy. Unlike amniocentesis, women who have had a transcervical CVS procedure tend to experience some bleeding through the vagina, particularly if the cervical os has been held with velsellum forceps to stabilise the cervix during the procedure.

Women should be warned, however, that persistent pain and heavy blood loss are a matter of concern, and should be reported to and monitored by maternity care staff. Checking for fetal viability with ultrasound can confirm if a pregnancy has ended and it is important that psychological support is offered to the woman and her partner if this occurs. It is recommended that any pregnancy loss, regardless of gestation, should be treated as a loss. Other agencies can prove useful for couples who have experienced this. Some contact details are given in Chapter 2.

Table 10.2   Potential maternal and fetal complications that can arise following prenatal diagnosis

Maternal (fetal*)	Reason for complication
Sepsis*	Intrauterine infection acquired from organisms on the maternal abdomen or introduced by the operator (equipment/hands). This is rare but is potentially fatal both for mother and baby. Can result in chorioamnionitis
Haemorrhage* Haematoma*	Needle puncture can cause bleeding within uterine wall, placenta or cord vessel Bleeding could result in a clot where puncture occurred. If in uterus, can cause contractions and within umbilical cord can cause vasospasm resulting in fetal anoxia
Embolisation*	An obstruction within the maternal uterine sinuses as a result of minute particles of deciduas within amniotic fluid. Extremely rare
Sensitisation*	Fetal blood that enters the maternal circulation as a consequence of needling can result in the production of maternal antibodies
Uterine contractions	As a consequence of either piercing the uterus or causing bruising to the sensitive muscle fibres
Maternal death*	Very rare but could be attributable to sepsis, haemorrhage or amniotic embolisation

TRANSPORTATION OF SAMPLE

Either the doctor or midwife attending the woman should, as matter of good practice, immediately place fluid or tissue samples obtained from amniocentesis, CVS and cordocentesis within an appropriate container. Personal details, including full name, residence, date of birth and hospital numbers should be obtained from the midwife and clearly documented on both the container and the laboratory form. Where cordocentesis is performed and fetal blood obtained, the samples should be gently shaken to avoid clotting. The healthcare professional should ensure that the laboratory form and containers clearly indicate that the sample is fetal in origin and that the specimen is not maternal blood.

INHERITED CONDITIONS

Understanding procedures and processes

This chapter has described a variety of prenatal diagnostic methods that can inform couples about the health of their baby. Couples may be interested in learning how samples from amniocentesis, CVS or cordocentesis are tested within their local laboratory. It is helpful if midwives have a basic knowledge of laboratory procedures, so that they can answer any questions asked by the couple. Unless

information is accurate and presented in such a way that it can be readily assimilated, the woman and her partner may not understand the processes involved and may be unable to make decisions which reflect their beliefs. Scanty, misleading information could cause them to make wrong choices, which they may regret for future weeks, months or years. Hence, it is important that midwives supporting women undergoing prenatal investigations be up to date with local policies and information around this specialist field, and give accurate advice to women and couples within their care.

Understanding patterns of inheritance

Women and couples today are often interested not just in the technology of prenatal testing and diagnosis, but also in the physiology of intrauterine life and the causes of abnormality. Although clinical genetic teams and obstetricians who specialise in fetal medicine have traditionally delivered prenatal diagnostic test results, midwives are becoming more involved as technology is advancing. Ideally, midwives should complement and support the role of the obstetrician or clinical geneticist whose responsibility it is to provide accurate information in relation to risk estimation, diagnosis and follow up of an existing or newly diagnosed disorder. Primarily, the midwife's function is to provide basic information or reiterate that provided by specialists, to ensure that what has been said has been understood. The midwife is there to identify where there are difficulties, as sometimes the information presented is overwhelming, and where appropriate clarify concerns or refer women back for further counselling. Midwives therefore require a basic awareness and understanding of the concepts of genetics and prenatal testing, so that they can prepare women and support them before and during testing and after results are generated. Thus, any midwife caring for women undergoing prenatal screening or diagnosis should possess the skills and information needed to explain the basic patterns of inheritance. This will help to prepare women and their partners for the more detailed information which may be required should a test result generate unexpected findings.

The human chromosome complement

Within each human cell lies the nucleus and within this structure are the chromosomes, which contain the most basic structure within the human body. Deoxyribonucleic acid (DNA) is a molecule containing the information which gives us our characteristics, inherited from our parents. The DNA contains over 100 000 genes which provide instructions that can influence our health and wellbeing throughout life.

Human cells contain two of almost every gene (diploid). The human karyotype consists of 22 pairs of autosomes and two further chromosomes which as well as having the same function as the autosomes have a specific task of establishing the sex of an individual. These are known as the sex chromosomes. In females there are two X chromosomes and in males one X and one Y chromosome. Thus, when fertilisation occurs between the egg of the mother and sperm of the father, each contributes one autosome and one sex chromosome, which result in a new life bearing a complement of 46 chromosomes. This is written as 46XX for a normal female or 46XY for a normal male.

The laboratory identifies each chromosome by its characteristic size and banding pattern when stained in metaphase, the stage of mitosis in which replicated chromosomes align at the centre (spindle) of the cell.

Make-up of a chromosome

On an initial glance, it may appear that a chromosome is shaped just like a long piece of string. In fact, the chromosome consists of three parts: an upper portion is known as the 'p' arm and the lower is called the 'q' arm; connecting both is the centromere, the point of attachment for the p and q portions of the chromosome.

Chromosomes 13, 14, 15, 21 and 22 are known as 'acrocentric' because the centromere is placed further towards one end. They are made up of a small amount of material in the p arm and more material in the q arm. These are the chromosomes that can result in a Robertsonian translocation, which will be discussed later.

Autosomal dominant pattern of inheritance

On each chromosome and its partner chromosome is a gene responsible for enzyme activity. The chromosome pair (allele) together determines the character of the individual (hair, eye and skin colour, physical features and so on). Some genes need only be present in one chromosome, rather than two, before they are expressed and are therefore called 'dominant' as shown in Figure 10.8. Autosomal dominant conditions can affect both males and females and are usually transmitted through affected family members. Examples of dominant conditions are shown in Box 10.5. An autosomal dominant condition may not manifest until late in the individual's life and signs and symptoms of the condition may vary from individual to individual. It is known that the dominant gene may not always express itself completely and as a consequence the individual leads a healthy normal life. People may be totally unaware of having an autosomal dominant gene condition, and it is only when signs and symptoms affect another family member that the condition is revealed through genetic testing.

Autosomal recessive pattern of inheritance

For an individual to be affected by an autosomal recessive condition, two altered genes have to come together, one from the mother and one from the father. The parents, although they are carriers of the altered gene, do not experience signs or symptoms of the disorder. Figure 10.9 illustrates that in each pregnancy, the parents would always have a one in four chance of having an affected offspring. The

Dominant inheritance

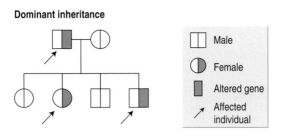

Figure 10.8 Autosomal dominant pattern of inheritance.

Recessive inheritance

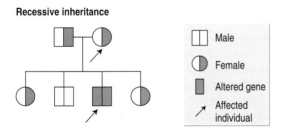

Figure 10.9 Autosomal recessive pattern of inheritance. Note that there is a 1 in 4 chance of an affected child.

conditions that are shown in Box 10.6, including some that are inborn errors of metabolism, screened for on the newborn blood spot card (Guthrie), are all recessively inherited. Recently, across England, a universal sickle cell screening programme was introduced so that babies could be tested for the disorder. Similarly, antenatal sickle cell and thalassaemia screening was introduced within some maternity services as finding the presence of these disorders can identify couples at risk and early diagnosis can be made in couples who are found to be carriers.

Where prenatal diagnosis confirms positive results, proactive planning can ensure that as soon as the baby is born, the appropriate treatment can be put into place.

X-linked patterns of inheritance

As previously mentioned, as well as inheriting 44 autosomes during conception, we also receive from our parents a pair of sex chromosomes, which brings the complement up to 46 chromosomes. However, sometimes an individual will be affected by an X-linked disorder as a consequence of an altered gene on one of the X chromosomes.

X-linked disorders manifest in males who, on their one and only X chromosome, have inherited from their 'healthy' mother a copy of the altered gene. Because they have two X chromosomes, women are not affected by X-linked disorders, since the healthy X chromosome dominates the faulty one. Thus women are unaffected carriers and males in the family can be affected by the condition as shown in Figure 10.10. Where a woman is pregnant with a male fetus, there is a 50% chance of the pregnancy being affected by disorders such as haemophilia, Duchenne muscular dystrophy and others as listed in Box 10.7.

Aneuploidy

Aneuploidy is a term used in clinical genetics to describe an alteration of the chromosomes. It is where someone has one or a few chromosomes above or below the normal complement of 46, which can be detrimental to the health and well-being of the fetus. Abnormal ultrasound findings can in some instances be attributed to aneuploidy depending on whether the abnormality is part of a chromosomal syndrome or disorder. The most

X-linked inheritance inheritance

Healthy female carrier

☐☐	Male
◐	Female
▉	Altered gene
↗	Affected individual

Healthy female carrier Affected male Non-carrier/ not affected

Figure 10.10   X-linked inheritance. Males are always affected, whilst females are healthy carriers.

Box 10.7   X-linked recessive disorders

- Becker's muscular dystrophy
- Colour blindness
- Duchenne muscular dystrophy
- Fabry's disease
- Haemophilia
- Hunter's syndrome

---

common form of aneuploidy is Down's syndrome, where instead of the typical 46 chromosomes there are 47. Down's syndrome can arise in a variety of ways, the most common being non-dysjunction trisomy 21.

Non-dysjunction trisomy 21

Non-dysjunctional trisomy, the commonest way in which Down's syndrome occurs, happens during meiosis (the cell division process that eggs and sperm undergo which halves the chromosome number from 46 to 23) when an extra copy of chromosome 21 (usually maternal in origin) results in each cell containing 47, instead of 46, chromosomes. Although this can happen at any age, there is a strong association with advanced maternal age.

Mosaic trisomy 21

People with this condition have mixed cell lines (the presence of two or more chromosome patterns within the cells), some having a normal set of chromosomes and others having trisomy 21. Physically they will have some of the typical features of Down's syndrome, but these may be quite subtle.

Robertsonian translocation

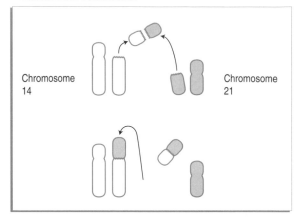

Figure 10.11   Robertsonian translocation.

Robertsonian chromosomal translocation

A translocation refers to the transfer of genetic material between one chromosome and another. A reciprocal translocation occurs when a break occurs in two chromosomes and the segments are exchanged to form new derivative chromosomes.

The Robertsonian translocation is another way in which Down's syndrome can occur, happening in about 5% of cases. It comes about when two chromosomes fuse together end to end, as shown in Figure 10.11 Either parent may carry a translocation but may be completely unaware as they have the correct amount of chromosomal material. Problems arise when they have children as the parent may pass on the two fused chromosomes as well as the normal chromosome, resulting in the pregnancy having three copies of chromosome 21.

LABORATORY INVESTIGATIONS

Scientists working within cytogenetic and molecular genetic laboratory services can perform a variety of laboratory investigations on prenatal diagnostic samples, which can give women and their partners information about the chromosomal or genetic constitution of their unborn child.

Depending on the indication for the diagnostic test, liquor, placental tissue or cord blood can be sent either to a cytogenetic or molecular genetic laboratory. These are usually placed within the same building. The sample may be spilt between the laboratories when more than one type of analysis is required for a particular condition.

TYPES OF ANALYSIS

Three different types of analysis are available to provide information about chromosomal and genetic variations within the fetus. All of these tests can be used on pregnancy samples. However, some laboratories have only recently begun to offer this range of choice. As screening for antenatal conditions advances, particularly where screening for Down's syndrome has been advocated as a universal screening programme,[29,50,52] traditional methods of karyotyping, used for the past 20 years, are being replaced by more advanced and rapid methods of analysis. These can provide women and their partners with results more quickly. The next part of the chapter explains and discusses advantages and disadvantages of these methods.

Methods of cytogenetic and molecular analysis include:

- Standard culture or karyotype
- Fluorescence in situ hybridisation (FISH)
- Quantitative fluorescence-polymerase chain reaction (QF-PCR).

Karyotyping

The standard culture, otherwise known as karyotyping, is commonly used to diagnose Down's syndrome, other trisomies, balanced and unbalanced translocations and the sex of the fetus. It involves counting all chromosomes and examining their structure and shape. Amniotic fluid, placental tissue or cord blood can be used for this method. However, for the purposes of explaining the test, amniotic fluid will be used as an example.

On receipt of the sample, the fluid is put into sterile tubes and centrifuged (Figure 10.12) to collect the amniocytes (fetal cells). These cells are

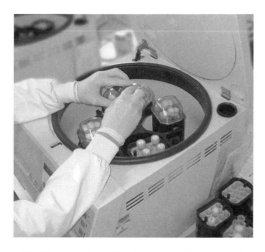

Figure 10.12   Amniotic fluid samples being put into a centrifuge to separate fetal cells from amniotic fluid.

then mixed with a culture medium and a drop is placed onto each of a few petri dishes as shown in Figure 10.13. The cells are then grown for 7–10 days in an incubator. At around day 10 or 11, the cells are harvested, put onto slides and then stained and analysed under a microscope (Fig. 10.14). Figure 10.15 shows cells at the metaphase stage of division when they should have 46 chromosomes. One of the metaphases is selected and a karyotype prepared.

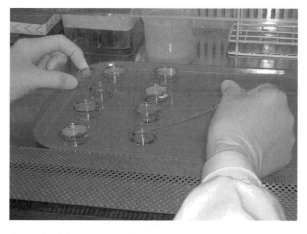

Figure 10.13   Preparation of fetal cells for incubation (taken from amniocentesis sample).

Although the full karyotype guarantees to detect non-trisomy abnormalities as well as trisomic conditions, the main disadvantages is the longer wait for results compared with new rapid methods of analysis.

As shown in Figure 10.16 a normal karyotype is one with 46 chromosomes altogether, including the two sex chromosomes. The chromosomes are organised in pairs in relation to shape and size, with the largest being labelled as chromosome 1 and the smallest chromosome 22. The two sex chromosomes are in addition to this.

More rapid diagnostic techniques

The demand for rapid analysis and reporting of prenatal diagnostic samples is increasing as early results allow early intervention, give women more time to consider their options, and offer an earlier opportunity for medical termination if desired. From receipt of a sample, both FISH and QF-PCR are able to give women results within 48 hours, thus providing reassurance more quickly for women with negative results.

Fluorescence in situ hybridisation (FISH)

FISH is specifically designed to identify trisomies 13, 18 and 21 and any sex chromosome abnormalities. In simple terms, FISH uses coloured DNA probes that attach to specific regions of the chromosomes in fetal cells so that the cells can be analysed with a microscope. The DNA probes, which have different fluorescent dyes, are mixed with the fetal cells and attach to the chromosomes by a process called hybridisation. Because of their different labels, they can be used to detect more than one condition at the same time.

The mixture of DNA probes and fetal cells is placed on a slide and can be analysed after 24 hours. The number of spots in each cell is counted to establish if the expected number are present for chromosomes 13, 18 and 21, and for the X and Y chromosomes, or if there is an abnormality. The colour and number of fluorescent dots determines the diagnosis of trisomies 13, 18 and 21, and any sex chromosome abnormalities. An example is shown in Figure 10.17, where A shows two red signals for trisomy 21 (normal) and two green signals for trisomy 13 (normal), and B shows 3 red

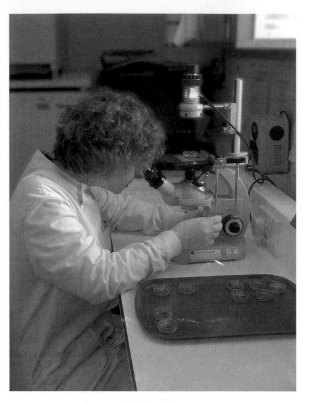

Figure 10.14   Checking fetal cells around days 10–11.

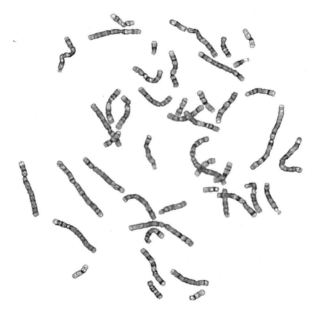

Figure 10.15   Microscope image of fetal cells in metaphase.

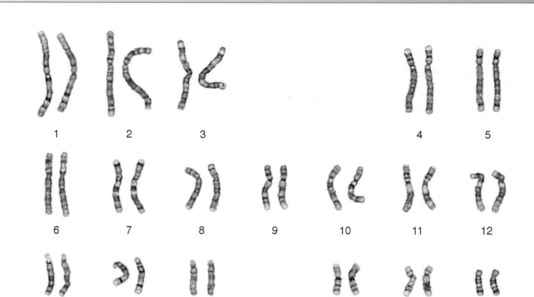

1	2	3		4	5
6	7	8	9	10	11	12
13	14	15		16	17	18
19	20		21	22	x	y

Figure 10.16   Normal karyotype (46 chromosomes).

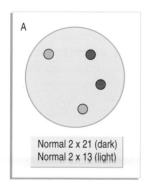

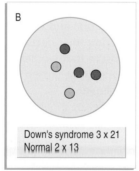

A

Normal 2 x 21 (dark)
Normal 2 x 13 (light)

B

Down's syndrome 3 x 21
Normal 2 x 13

Figure 10.17   Fluorescence in situ hybridisation (FISH). Analysis for trisomy 13 (Patau's syndrome) and 21 (Down's syndrome). Note that in A just two red and two green dots are present, indicative of a normal result, while in B the three red dots are indicative of Down's syndrome.

signals for trisomy 21 (abnormal – indicates Down's syndrome) and two green signals (normal) for trisomy 13.

FISH has been extensively validated as a reliable method of analysis; however, it is an expensive option as the process requires more resources and time than the standard culture technique.

Quantitative fluorescence-polymerase chain reaction (QF-PCR)

The second rapid technique for the diagnosis of trisomies 13, 18, 21 and abnormality of the sex chromosomes is QF-PCR. This is a rapid and robust technology that is highly automated, requiring fewer staff than the procedure for full karyotyping, and again involves the use of fluorescent technology. DNA is extracted from the fetal cells and then multiplied in concentration and labelled with fluorescent dyes to enable analysis. A sequencer measures specific regions on the DNA molecule with the results being displayed graphically on a computer screen as a series of peaks. To ensure the results are accurate, at least four different fragments for each chromosome are analysed.

Like FISH, QF-PCR has been extensively validated and requires only small amounts of DNA for analysis; however, it is much less troublesome than FISH in terms of laboratory handling and service management. Heavily blood-stained samples can interfere with analysis so it is important that operators avoid 'bloody taps' during needling procedures.

SOME CAUTIONS

Although these two technologies have the advantage of rapid reporting time, they have the disadvantage of only being able to diagnose four specific abnormalities compared with the standard karyotype, which is able to diagnose a spectrum of disorders.

It is imperative when discussing FISH and QF-PCR that midwives ensure that couples are aware that only a specific number of conditions can be diagnosed. If a karyotype is to be carried out as well as rapid testing, the midwife must ensure that consent has been given by the couple for this, so that they are aware that unexpected conditions may be found. It is important that midwives ensure that the laboratory request form is properly completed, stating the indication for diagnosis and the specific tests required. This should also be documented in the maternal and hospital notes.

Women and their partners also need to know that rapid techniques, like other technologies, have their limitations. It should be explained that blood-stained samples cannot be processed and occasionally a result cannot be generated. Women undergoing karyotype analysis for aneuploidy also need to be aware that genetic disorders and small deletions (microdeletions) will not be assessed.

CONCLUSION

Prenatal diagnosis is here to stay so long as antenatal screening remains driven by the desire for society to know as much as possible about intrauterine health. Controversy exists around this field of medical practice as the potential for eradicating illness is through the process of medical termination; however, whatever choices women and their partners face, healthcare professionals should not be there to judge but to support them as they face their dilemmas. Midwives have much to offer within this realm of practice, and can adapt and develop the same skills they use to support a woman in normal pregnancy to support women undergoing high-risk pregnancies.

Key Practice Points

- Midwives should be knowledgeable with up to date information about prenatal testing so that they can provide women and their partners with accurate information.
- Midwives should have an understanding of the advantages and disadvantages of invasive tests and how these can affect the woman's physical and psychological wellbeing.
- Women and their partners should be given both oral and written information to aid them during their decision-making. Midwives should ensure that women and their partners are made aware that testing is an option but not an obligation.
- Midwives should ensure that abnormal results generated from prenatal diagnosis are dealt with swiftly in order to reduce the distress and upset for the woman and her partner.

References

1. Gupton A, Heaman M, Ashcroft T. Bed rest from the perspective of the high-risk pregnant woman. Journal of Obstetric Gynecologic and Neonatal Nursing 1997; 26(4):423–430.
2. Maloni JA, Ponder M. Fathers' experience of their partners' antepartum bed rest. Journal of Nursing Scholarship 1997; 29(2):183–188.

3. Heaman M, Gupton A. Perceptions of bed-rest by women with high-risk pregnancies: a comparison between home and hospital. Birth 1998; 25(4):252–258.

4. Maloni JA, Kane JH, Suen LJ, Wang KK. Dysphoria among high-risk pregnant hospitalised women on bed rest. Nursing Research 2002; 512:92–99.

5. Thornburg P. 'Waiting' as experienced by women hospitalised during the antepartum period. MCN American Journal of Maternal Child Nursing 2002; 27(4):245–248.

6. Kirwan DM. Real voices: the search for silent witnesses. Women's experiences of haemolytic antibodies in pregnancy. MPhil Thesis 2004.

7. Buckley S. Prenatal diagnosis—technological triumph or Pandora's box? MIDIRS Midwifery Digest 2005; 15(1):7–14.

8. Niven CA. Psychological care for families: before, during and after birth. Oxford: Butterworth Heinemann; 1992.

9. Kempson E. Informing health consumers: a review of consumer health information needs and services. London: College of Health; 1987.

10. Kohner N. Understanding and being understood: Introduction and Module 1. Health care relationships. Antenatal Screening Project. A Welsh Assembly Government/Velindre NHS Trust Project. Cardiff: 1998.

11. Royal College of Obstetricians and Gynaecologists. Amniocentesis and chorionic villus sampling. Guideline No.8. RCOG; London: 2005.

12. Kirwan DM, Walkinshaw SA. Amniocentesis and the specialist midwife: the developing role. The Practising Midwife 2000; 3(5):14–18.

13. Sutton A. Prenatal diagnosis: confronting the ethical issues. London: The Linacre Centre; 1990.

14. Whelton J. The midwife and foetal medicine. Nursing 1990; 4:1.

15. Garrett C, Charlton L. Difficult decisions in prenatal diagnosis. In: Abramsky L, Chapple J. Prenatal diagnosis: the human side. London: Chapman and Hall 1984; 86–105.

16. Lambl D. Ein seltener Fall von Hydramnios. Zentralbl Gynaekol 1881; 5:329.

17. Schatz F. Eine besondere Art von ein seitiger Polyhydramnioc mit anderseitiger Oligohydramnie bei Zwillingen. Arch Gynaekol 1882; 19:329.

18. Menees TD, Miller JD, Holly LE. Amniography: preliminary report. American Journal Roentgenol Radium Therapy 1930; 24:363.

19. Aburel ME. Le déclenchement du travail par injections intraamniotique de serum sale hypertonique. Gynecol Obstet 1937; 36:398.

20. Bevis DCA. The antenatal prediction of haemolytic disease of the newborn. Lancet 1952; 1(8):395–398.

21. Walker A. Liquor amnii studies in the prediction of haemolytic disease of the newborn. British Medical Journal 1957; 2(5041):376–378.

22. Fuchs F, Riis P. Antenatal sex determination. Nature 1956;117:330.

23. Steele MW, Breg WR. Chromosome analysis of human amniotic fluid cells. Lancet 1966; 1(7434):383–385.

24. Valenti C, Shutta EJ, Kehaty T. Prenatal diagnosis of Down's syndrome. Lancet 1968; 2(7561):220.

25. Nadler HL. Antenatal detection of hereditary disorders. Paediatrics 1968; 42:912.

26. Brock DJH, Sutcliffe RG. Alpha-fetoprotein in the antenatal diagnosis of anencephaly and spina bifida. Lancet 1972; 2:197–199.

27. Nicolaides K, Brizot M de L, Patel F, Snijders R. Comparison of chorionic villus sampling and amniocentesis for fetal karyotyping at 10–13 weeks' gestation. Lancet 1994; 344(8920):435–439.

28. The Canadian Early and Midtrimester Amniocentesis Trial (CEMAT) Group. Randomized trial to assess safety and fetal outcome of early and midtrimester amniocentesis. Lancet 1998; 351(9098):242–247.

29. UK National Screening Committee. Testing for Down's syndrome in pregnancy: choosing whether to have the tests is an important decision, for you and your baby. Oxford: UKNSC; 2004.

30. Crandon AJ, Peel JR. Amniocentesis with and without ultrasound guidance. British Journal of Obstetrics and Gynaecology 1979; 86:1–3.

31. Romero R, Jeanty P, Reece EA, et al. Sonographically monitored amniocentesis to decrease intra-operative complications. Obstetrics and Gynaecology 1985; 65:426–430.

32. De Crespigny LC, Robinson HP. Amniocentesis; a comparison of monitored versus blind needle insertion. Australian New Zealand Journal of Obstetrics and Gynaecology 1986; 26:124–128.

33. Squier M, Chamberlaine P, Zaiwealla Z, et al. Five cases of brain injury following amniocentesis in mid-term pregnancy. Dev Med Child Neurol 2000; 42:554–560.

34. Nicolini U. Invasive techniques of prenatal diagnosis. Current Obstetrics and Gynaecology 1992; 2:77–84.

35. Mohr J. Foetal genetic diagnosis: development of techniques for early sampling of foetal cells. Acta Pathologica Microbiolabic Scandinavia 1968; 73:7377.

36. Department of Obstetrics and Gynaecology. Tietung Hospital of Anshan Iron and Steel Company, Anshan, China. Fetal sex prediction by sex chromatin of chorionic villi cells during early pregnancy. Chinese Medical Journal 1975; 1:117–126.

37. Firth HV, Boyd PA, Chamberlain P, et al. Severe limb abnormalities after chorionic villus sampling at 55–66 days' gestation. Lancet 1991; 337(8744):762–763.

38. Burton BK, Schulz CK, Burd LI. Limb anomalies associated with chorionic villus sampling. Obstetrics and Gynaecology 1992; 79:726–730.

39. Burton BK, Schulz CK, Burd LI. Limb anomalies associated with chorionic villus sampling. Obstet Gynecol 1992; 79(5, Part 1):726–730.

40. Dolk H, Bertrand F, Lechat MF. Chorionic villus sampling and limb abnormalities. Lancet 1992; 339(8797):876–877.

41. Liu DTY. Analysis of limb reduction defects after chorionic villus sampling. Lancet 1994; 343(8905):1069–1071.

42. Rodeck C. Fetoscopy and chorion biopsy. Current Therapy in Neonatal-Perinatal Medicine 1985–1986:84–89.

43. Green JM. Women's experiences of diagnostic tests. In: Abramskey L, Chapple J. Prenatal diagnosis: the human side. London: Chapman and Hall 1994; 37–53.

44. Daffos F, Capella-Pavlovsky M, Forestier F. Fetal blood sampling via the umbilical cord using a needle guided by ultrasound. Report of 66 cases. Prenatal Diagnosis 1985; 3:271–277.

45. Freda VJ, Adamson K. Exchange transfusion in utero. American Journal of Obstetrics and Gynaecology 1964; 89:817–821.

46. Rodeck C, Campbell S. Umbilical insertion as a source of pure fetal blood for prenatal diagnosis. Lancet 1979; 1(8129):1244–1245.

47. Antsaklis AI, Papantoniou NE, Mesogitis SA, et al. Cardiocentesis: an alternative method of fetal blood sampling for the prenatal diagnosis of haemoglobinopathies. Obstetrics and Gynaecology 1992; 79:630–633.

48. Walkinshaw SA. What happens when a sensitising event goes undetected? A case for routine antenatal prophylaxis. Anti-D prophylaxis the way forward (Bulletin). Bio Products Laboratory Hertfordshire: Haymarket Publications; 2000.

49. National Institute for Clinical Excellence (NICE). Technology Appraisal No. 41. Guidance on the use of routine antenatal anti-D prophylaxis for RhD-negative women. London: NICE; 2002.

50. National Institute for Clinical Excellence (NICE). Clinical Guideline 6. Antenatal care: routine care for the healthy pregnant woman. London: NICE; 2003.

51. Royal College of Obstetricians and Gynaecologists. Green Top Guideline. Use of anti-D immunoglobulin for Rh prophylaxis. London: RCOG; 2002.

52. UK National Screening Committee. Model of best practice. Oxford: NSC; 2003.

11

Assessment of fetal wellbeing

Lucy Kean

INTRODUCTION

Antenatal care is the major screening tool used for assessment of fetal wellbeing in the late second and third trimesters in the healthy pregnant woman. Various components of screening are now embedded within the NICE guideline on antenatal care[1] and should form a routine part of care. The NICE guideline only covers routine antenatal care of the low-risk woman, and therefore the value judgements midwives make on a case by case basis regarding risk also form a vital part of the assessment of fetal wellbeing. The challenge for antenatal care is to correctly identify women whose fetuses are developing problems, without subjecting a population of normal women to interventions which may lead on to further intervention and morbidity which may be unnecessary. It is a sad fact though, that stillbirth at or near term is commoner in the population of women deemed to be low risk than those at high risk, and that 50% of these fetuses will turn out to be growth restricted on post-mortem.[2] In a low-risk population, routine antenatal care will only detect between 17% and 25% of growth restricted fetuses.[3] Whether a consistent approach to screening for fetal wellbeing in a low-risk population will improve on this is still to be established.

FETAL ADAPTATION

In order to understand how tests for fetal wellbeing work, it is important to understand how a fetus adapts as it becomes compromised. The adaptive changes discussed here relate mainly to the fetus having to adapt to less than ideal placental perfusion.

Fetal movements (FM)

One of the earliest responses a fetus can make to poor placental perfusion is simply to conserve energy by moving less.[4] It is apparent that early changes in fetal movements are sometimes very subtle, e.g. a slight prolongation of sleep phases, but as placental perfusion becomes more compromised a measurable diminution in fetal activity can often be seen. A reduction in the amount of time the fetus spends breathing is also apparent.

Growth

As placental nutrition fails, the fetus attempts to conserve growth in vital organs. These include the brain, heart and adrenal glands. The usual pattern of fetal weight gain with glycogen stored in the fetal liver and subcutaneous fat deposition will stop and if placental nutrition continues to be poor, the fetus will use up stored glycogen. This leads to a recognisable pattern of growth restriction termed 'late onset' or 'asymmetrical' growth restriction, where the head circumference measurements are normal but the abdominal circumference (which is measured at the level of the fetal liver) is on a lower centile (see Fig. 11.1). This must not be confused with the opposite, where head measurements are small but abdominal growth is conserved, as this has an entirely different set of potential pathologies.

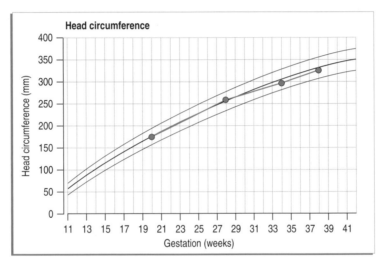

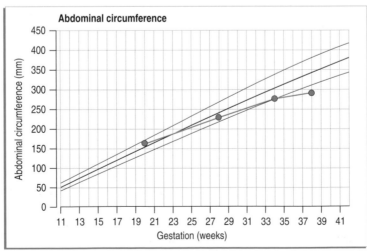

Figure 11.1 Growth chart showing late onset (asymmetrical) growth restriction. A. Head circumference; B. Abdominal circumference.

Vascular adaptation

The mechanism the fetus uses to divert critical nutrition and oxygenated blood to vital organs is its ability to alter vascular distribution. The fetus can reduce blood flow to organs such as the kidneys and gut by as much as 80% if necessary. It compensates by vasodilatation of the vessels in the target organs such as the brain.[5] If renal blood flow is severely curtailed, fetal urine output will decline, whilst fetal swallowing movements may be maintained. This leads to a fall in the liquor volume (which is almost exclusively fetal urine by this stage of pregnancy). The diversion of blood flow from the fetal gut can mean that after birth the gut is relatively under-perfused and if this is severe the gut will be unable to tolerate oral feeding until blood flow has been re-established and recovery occurs. This can take 48 hours or longer in the most compromised fetuses. If compromise is combined with prematurity, enteral feeding in the early stages can lead to necrotising enterocolitis. The neonatologists are thus often circumspect about feeding orally in the early stages when there has been evidence of vascular redistribution.

Cerebral blood flow increases to allow delivery of vital resources to the growing fetal brain. This adaptation can be sought as part of the diagnosis of fetal compromise. Only if placental perfusion becomes critically poor will central nervous system changes be seen. These include a blunting of the sympathetic and parasympathetic response, leading to a loss of the normal fetal heart rate variability; and if hypoxia is developing, chemoreceptors may be triggered, causing shallow decelerations of the fetal heart rate. The fetus will usually also have increased its heart rate slightly, in order to maximise perfusion of the placenta. However, it is unusual for the heart rate to move above the normal range of 160 beats per minute (bpm). A loss of variability has been shown to occur when the fetal pH drops below 7.2. Accelerations also disappear at this stage.[6]

SCREENING TESTS FOR FETAL WELLBEING

These can be divided into initial screening and further tests. Initial screening includes identification of maternal conditions that have a fetal impact (such as smoking, pre-eclampsia, severe anaemia), asking about and reporting of fetal movements, abdominal palpation and symphysis fundal height (SFH) measurement. Further tests of fetal wellbeing include cardiotocography, ultrasound for aspects of fetal wellbeing, Doppler evaluation and, very rarely, other invasive tests to look for specific diagnoses, such as fetal anaemia or chromosomal disease.

Identification of maternal risk

This is the first screening test applied to pregnant women and is first done at the booking visit but is updated on each subsequent visit. It is an integral part of antenatal care and is rarely thought of as a screening test, but is a vital part of our ability to screen those women who are already or are becoming at increased risk of fetal problems. The booking visit identifies factors that may lead to referral to an obstetrician and the hospital taking the lead role. This may include maternal factors such as pre-existing disease, e.g. hypertension or diabetes, which lead to hospital led care, or factors such as smoking, which increase the fetal risk, but for which hospital referral may not be necessary. The list of factors, which can impact on the fetus from the booking visit, is long and is covered well in the introductory chapter of the NICE guideline on antenatal care.[1]

Reassessment of maternal risk

Some reassessment of maternal risk is made at every antenatal visit. The blood pressure (BP) is measured and the urine tested. These are excellent screening tests for the development of hypertension and proteinuria. Of course, as with any screening test there will be the inevitable false positives and negatives, but repeated testing is usually able to distinguish mothers who are developing problems from those who are not. Sometimes the picture can only be clarified by more rigorous investigation, such as 24-hour urine collection or repeated BP analysis. Urinalysis may reveal glycosuria. The presence of glucose in the urine is a poor indicator for developing gestational diabetes (GDM) as many women with the condition will never have glycosuria and most women with glycosuria do not have GDM.[1] However, some units still test for this and if glucose is present on two occasions a random blood sugar should be performed. If this is greater than 6.1, a formal glucose tolerance test should be organised. Interestingly, a random sugar taken in the mid-afternoon appears to show the best sensitivity.[1] Uncorrected severe anaemia is associated with growth restriction and preterm birth. The routine screening of haemoglobin at booking, 28 and 34 weeks is designed to detect those mothers who will benefit from iron supplementation.

Assessment of fetal risk

An assessment of fetal risk will be made at booking based on those factors that are available at that time. The most important factors will include:

- Maternal disease such as diabetes, antiphospholipid syndrome (see Ch. 4)
- Maternal age
- Maternal lifestyle (smoking, alcohol, drugs)
- Maternal characteristics (obesity, severely underweight)
- Previous obstetric history (recurrent or late miscarriage, growth restriction, preterm labour, pre-eclampsia)
- Red cell antibodies.

Maternal disease can affect the fetus by direct metabolic or chronic hypoxic effects (such as diabetes or cystic fibrosis) or by causing a placental disease which then reduces fetal reserve, such as antiphospholipid syndrome, hypertension and insulin dependent diabetes. Mothers conceiving for the first time at a very young age and a later age (in particular under 18 or over 40) are at increased risk for pre-eclampsia, intrauterine growth restriction (IUGR) and preterm delivery.

Smoking continues to be a leading risk factor for growth restriction and stillbirth. Mothers using alcohol in large amounts and illicit drugs are also at risk. Women who are significantly overweight (body mass index (BMI) >35) are more likely to suffer a stillbirth than women of normal weight. It is certainly clear that IUGR is much more difficult to diagnose clinically in these women and it is likely that the higher incidence of gestational diabetes also contributes. In underweight women (BMI <18) the major risks are of IUGR and preterm delivery.

A past obstetric history of recurrent or late miscarriage increases the risk of preterm labour, IUGR and a repeat event. Any woman who has delivered a baby at term weighing less than 2.5 kg should have increased surveillance for fetal growth. Women who have previously delivered prematurely require an individualised assessment of risk and a strategy for surveillance based on that assessment. The same is true for women who have previously developed pre-eclampsia, as the antenatal care for a woman with previous severe early onset pre-eclampsia will differ radically from that needed for a woman who developed mild late onset disease in a first pregnancy but who had a trouble-free second pregnancy.

The pattern of fetal assessment performed as part of antenatal care will be based on the maternal and fetal risk factors. Where no increased risk is identified, antenatal care will proceed as defined in the NICE guideline.[1] At each visit, a reassessment of fetal risk will be made.

Reassessment of fetal risk

Fetal risk is reassessed at every visit as part of the maternal risk assessment for pre-eclampsia and GDM and is also separately assessed by a number of screening tests, including asking about fetal movements, abdominal palpation and symphysis fundal height measurement.

Fetal movements

Most pregnant women begin to feel fetal movements from 18–20 weeks' gestation. Ultrasound studies show that movements become more frequent during the afternoon and into the early evening. Women perceive movements more easily when lying than sitting or standing.[4] As pregnancy progresses in the third trimester, kicks become replaced by stretches and rolls and women may report a change in the type of fetal activity. However, as term approaches the fetus does not become less active and the total number of movements should be sustained. Hiccoughs are common especially between 28 and 32 weeks and have no pathological significance. Also, no consistent pathology has ever been attributable to an increase in fetal movements.

Fetal movement may be assessed formally, by means of counting and recording, or informally, by asking questions regarding movements and asking mothers to report changes in the fetal movements. Formal counting is limited by the fact that mothers report enormously varied ranges when questioned about fetal movements. The perception of fetal movements can be altered by:

- Maternal habitus
- Placental site (up to 28 weeks)
- Fetal position/presentation
- Maternal activity.

Pathological causes of reduced movements include:

- Sedative drugs (codeine, opiates, alcohol)
- Reduced placental perfusion
- Fetal anaemia
- Neurological abnormality
- Oligo- or polyhydramnios
- Fetal infection.

Some healthy fetuses will reportedly move less than 10 times each day whilst other mothers will say that their baby moves all the time. Formal fetal movement counting was not shown to reduce perinatal mortality compared with an informal approach in one large randomised study.[7] Perhaps the most important messages that we should give are:

- Fetuses do not become less active as they near term. The change in type of movement may mean that mothers need to concentrate more on this aspect of their baby in order to be sure that the baby is indeed moving normally.
- A change in fetal movements should be reported. It is illogical to ask a woman whose baby routinely moves 80–100 times each day to count to 10 movements and then not to worry. A reduction from 80 to 20 movements for this baby is a potentially worrying sign and should be reported.

Any woman who reports a reduction in fetal movements must be assessed as a matter of urgency. The methods of assessment are discussed below under further testing.

Abdominal palpation and assessment of fetal growth

Until 36 weeks there is no value in abdominal palpation for fetal presentation, unless delivery is likely. Some women find palpation uncomfortable, especially the assessment of the presenting part and engagement. However, an assessment of fetal size and liquor volume can be made by measurement of the symphysis fundal height (SFH). A reduction in fetal size or liquor volume, or both, may be detected if care is taken in the assessment. Whilst there are not good studies showing benefit of SFH measurement over routine palpation, the charting of measurements provides a clear guide for the next practitioner with regard to findings; and where care is often fragmented, this may improve the identification of IUGR in the healthy population. One large interventional study assessing the use of customised SFH charts (where maternal parameters are used to derive the chart) showed an increased detection of small and large for gestational age fetuses, without increasing the number of scans requested, in comparison to the usual care group.[8] The NICE guideline[1] now recommends that a formal measure of the SFH is made and recorded on an appropriate chart. It is important to plot the measurement as fundal height in centimetres is usually slightly less than the gestation in weeks and growth restriction is overdiagnosed if correct charts are not used (i.e. fundal height in cm should be 1–2 cm less than gestational age) (Fig. 11.2).

Referral for the small baby should be made when there has been a crossing of centiles, or a measurement is less than the 10th centile where there have been no other measurements made. It is important to look to see which centile the fetal abdominal circumference was on at the time of the detailed scan when the first measurement was plotted, as the centile for the SFH should be approximately the same.

Mothers will also become very anxious about a potentially large baby. If the SFH measurement is above the 90th centile, or centiles are being crossed, the only rational test to do is a blood sugar estimation, as the only intervention that may have benefit will be in mothers who are developing gestational diabetes. Ultrasound scanning is notoriously inaccurate in the larger fetus, and intervention such as induction of labour is of no proven benefit.

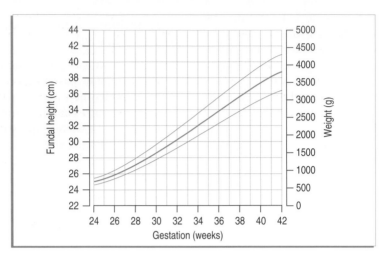

Figure 11.2 Symphysis fundal height chart.

Fetal heart auscultation

If fetal movements are felt during the examination, the only reason to listen to the fetal heart is to allow the mother to hear it also, and for this a hand held Doppler device is required. Very occasionally fetal arrhythmias are detected by routine auscultation, but much anxiety is also created when missed beats (which are generally benign) are heard. The fetal heart rate changes associated with placental compromise are not amenable to detection by auscultation, as the heart rate is usually within the normal range, and any decelerations are too shallow to be identified. Loss of variability is also unlikely to be detected.

Fetal arrhythmias will usually lead to a change in fetal movements and referral for this indication alone would be indicated.

Routine auscultation of the fetal heart is not recommended except where a mother requests this for reassurance.[1] In this case allowing the mother to hear the fetal heart herself is useful.

FURTHER TESTING FOR FETAL WELLBEING

Cardiotocography (CTG)

Antenatal cardiotocography was introduced following perceived benefits from intrapartum fetal heart rate monitoring. It is a tool that has been refined in many ways, including computerised analysis, but the major problem that this technology faces is that changes are usually a late event and that the reassurance derived from a normal CTG can only be for a very limited time. It is possible that the trial of fetal movement counting failed to show benefit not because fetal movement counting is not effective, but because the intervention used if fetal movements were reduced was CTG, which may not be good enough alone for this indication.[6] Some units have moved to a policy of ultrasound in addition to CTG in cases of reduced movements, to assess growth, liquor volume and, in some units, umbilical artery Doppler waveforms. The American College of Obstetricians and Gynaecologists recommends CTG plus amniotic fluid volume assessment but recognises that these recommendations are based on limited and inconsistent scientific evidence.[9] There are no trials to assess these increased methods of surveillance over and above standard CTG monitoring and large trials are needed before this strategy can be recommended.

The criteria for assessment of the CTG in the antenatal period are essentially the same as for intrapartum use, except that the lack of accelerations antenatally would be a worrying sign. CTG should not be performed at a gestation at which delivery would not be undertaken if fetal salvage was needed. Whilst 28 weeks has been used historically as a cut-off below which CTG was not utilised for fetal assessment, improvements in neonatal care mean that 26 weeks is now used in many units. Interpretation of the fetal heart rate at very early gestations is not as fraught as some would believe. Variability tends to be slightly less but accelerations will occur in the healthy fetus and accelerations remain hallmarks of fetal health. Persistent decelerations are worrying but must always be assessed in context. Where a very premature fetus has a non-reassuring antepartum CTG, a full fetal assessment by a senior clinician is warranted.

Cardiotocography is useful in the following scenarios:

- An initial test of fetal wellbeing when there is a reported problem such as reduced FM (very short-term reassurance)
- A means of ongoing assessment when mothers do not perceive fetal movements in a fetus that seems to be moving or has been tested in other ways and found to be healthy
- Monitoring of a fetus at risk where increased surveillance is required (e.g. a mother with pre-eclampsia who is an inpatient may have the fetus monitored once or twice each day, or a mother with diabetes, being monitored twice weekly as an outpatient).

Ultrasound assessment of fetal wellbeing

Ultrasound can be divided into its various components, each of which is targeted to assess whether there has been a fetal adaptive response.

Growth

Ultrasound is generally a good tool for assessing the under-growing fetus. It is much better at this than it is at assessment of the over-growing fetus. Routine ultrasound of low-risk women has never been shown to improve fetal outcomes; however, appropriately sized trials may clarify this, as these have never been performed.

Late onset (asymmetrical) growth restriction is usually of placental origin. It is characterised by reduced abdominal circumference when compared to head circumference (see Fig. 11.1). The implication is that the fetal reserves of glycogen have already been utilised to allow continued growth of key organs such as the brain. Reduced head, abdominal and femur measurements may point to

different pathologies. The commonest reason for the fetus to be small is simply that it is a small but healthy fetus (constitutionally small). This is often the case for mothers who are themselves small, or of Asian of Far Eastern origin. A customised growth chart can reduce the anxiety this finding can produce by taking into account the maternal factors that primarily influence growth. These include:

- Maternal weight
- Maternal height
- Parity
- Ethnic origin.

Customised growth charts are available via the website of the West Midlands Perinatal Epidemiology Unit (www.wmpho.org.uk).

When a fetus is thought to be smaller than expected despite consideration of maternal characteristics, a full survey of the fetus should be repeated. This is essential as other causes of growth restriction such as chromosomal disease or infection will need to be considered.

Diminished head growth in the presence of normal abdominal growth should also prompt a full fetal survey, as potential causes will include infection, or neurological and anatomical problems. Sometimes, particularly if the head is deep within the pelvis, the cause may simply be difficulty in accurately measuring the fetal head. It is important that the head circumference is used after 20 weeks, as head shape may vary, making the biparietal diameter less accurate.

Liquor volume

Liquor volume changes with gestation, peaking at 28 weeks (see Fig. 11.3). A reduction in liquor volume may occur for the following reasons:

- Fetal redistribution of blood flow away from the kidneys
- Rupture of membranes (though liquor volume can be measurably normal in some cases)
- Maternal dehydration, such as secondary to a viral gastroenteritis
- Fetal renal or urinary tract abnormalities.

The measurement of liquor volume forms an important part of the diagnosis of the potential problem. Sometimes it is the first sign of a placenta that is not functioning effectively.

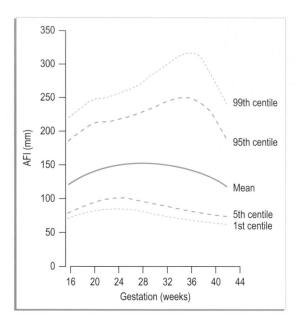

Figure 11.3 Amniotic fluid index (AFI).

Doppler analysis

The list of vessels that can be assessed by Doppler analysis grows year by year. Fetal vessels that provide the most information include:

- Umbilical artery
- Umbilical vein
- Middle cerebral artery
- Ductus venosus.

Doppler analysis of the umbilical artery is the only test that has been shown to improve fetal outcomes when used as a screening test in high-risk populations.[10] It is measured by identification of a free loop of cord and the measurement of the velocity of the red cells moving through the vessel. A ratio between the maximal systolic and the minimal diastolic readings is taken (see Fig. 11.4). Most units use either the pulsatility index (PI) or the resistance index (RI). The velocity of blood flow within the umbilical cord will be reduced if there is increased placental vascular resistance, but other factors such as fetal congenital heart problems can also give abnormal measurements. It is important to be aware that the umbilical artery Doppler measurements are not static. Diseases such as pre-eclampsia can show minor improvements and deteriorations over time as the disease

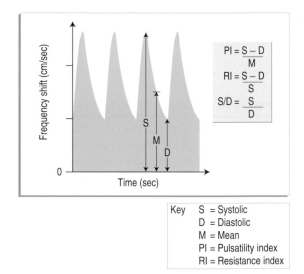

$$PI = \frac{S - D}{M}$$
$$RI = \frac{S - D}{S}$$
$$S/D = \frac{S}{D}$$

Key	S = Systolic
	D = Diastolic
	M = Mean
	PI = Pulsatility index
	RI = Resistance index

Figure 11.4 Doppler ratios. S: systolic; D: diastolic; M: mean; PI: pulsatility index; RI: resistance index.

relapses and remits. Single readings that are abnormal may need to be repeated in order to gain a full clinical picture. In general, when a placenta is failing the trend is for the index to be increased above the normal range, leading on to absent end diastolic velocity and if intervention does not occur,

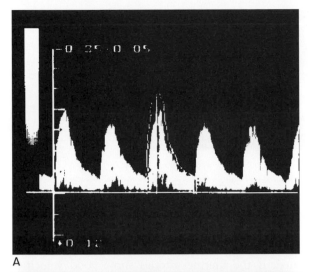

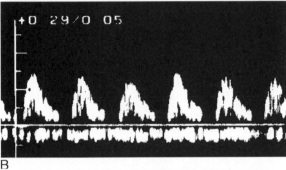

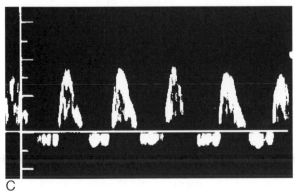

Figure 11.5 Sequentially worsening Dopplers. A: increased pulsatility index; B absent end diastolic velocity; C: reversed end diastolic velocity.

eventually to reversal of the end diastolic velocity (Fig. 11.5). The point at which intervention is undertaken (usually by delivery) will depend on the circumstances of the individual pregnancy. In general, a fetus showing reversed end diastolic velocity is likely to need delivery with 48 hours.

The middle cerebral artery (MCA) can be used to assess the fetus for two different pathologies:

■ Placental failure
■ Fetal anaemia.

As the placental function reduces, the fetus redistributes its vascular components to divert oxygenated blood primarily to its brain. The velocity of the blood flow within the fetal brain can be measured using the middle cerebral artery. This leads to a reduction below normal of the pulsatility index (i.e. increased velocity). This evidence would tend to corroborate a suspicion of placental dysfunction, e.g. where there is late onset (asymmetrical) growth restriction and an increase in umbilical artery Doppler measurements.

In the anaemic fetus the ratio of systolic and diastolic measurements within the MCA tends to stay within the normal range, but because the fetus has a much higher cardiac output due to the anaemia, the maximum velocity in this artery is increased. This is a useful non-invasive method of monitoring the potentially anaemic fetus, such as when there are rhesus antibodies.

Venous Dopplers

Venous Dopplers are used to fine tune assessment when delivery is becoming a possibility. They are of most value where the fetus is very immature and when even a few extra hours may confer benefit. Most clinicians would only move on to measure venous Dopplers when there is absent or reversed end diastolic velocity in the umbilical artery. Notching of the umbilical vein (Fig. 11.6) and reversal of the A wave in the ductus venosus are the two most useful measurements (Fig. 11.7). When these are seen, the fetus is highly likely to be becoming hypoxic and further prolongation of the pregnancy may not be of benefit.

Maternal uterine artery Doppler evaluation

This screening test is often undertaken when a woman has had a previous pregnancy affected by growth restriction or severe early onset pre-eclampsia. It is usually carried out between 22 and 24 weeks. The rationale is that the maternal uterine arteries should undergo vasodilatation in response to fetal trophoblast invasion. If trophoblast invasion is arrested before the level of the maternal spiral

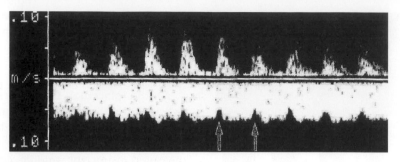

Figure 11.6   Notching umbilical vein.

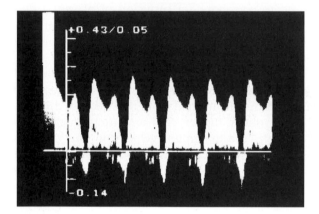

Figure 11.7   Reversed A wave in ductus venosus.

arteries, the mother retains a relatively high resistance uterine circulation. It is recognised that this occurs in some cases of pre-eclampsia and IUGR. In subsequent pregnancies, measurement of the uterine arteries can demonstrate whether conversion to a

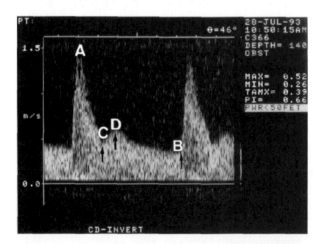

Figure 11.8   Uterine artery.

low resistance circulation has occurred. If this has not (notching is present in the uterine arteries, Fig. 11.8), then increased fetal and maternal surveillance is indicated. If the uterine arteries show good velocities with no notching, the risk of IUGR or pre-eclampsia developing subsequently becomes much smaller.

Biophysical profile

The biophysical profile was first defined by Manning in 1980.[11] It comprises a number of features that recognise the fetal adaptations made as the placental function declines. The initial definition scored either 0 or 2 for each parameter, but most units now use a score of 0 or 1, scoring the fetus out of 5. The parameters are defined in Table 11.1.

Each of the 5 components of the biophysical profile score does not have equal significance. Fetal breathing movements, amniotic fluid volume, and the CTG are the most important variables in assessment of wellbeing. For example, when the biophysical profile score is 1, the perinatal mortality varies from 428/1000 with only fetal movement present to 66/1000 if the CTG is reactive and all of the ultrasound parameters are absent. It is because of this finding that some have suggested that evaluation by CTG and amniotic fluid may replace the complete score.[9]

Only four randomised trials evaluating 2839 patients have compared the fetal biophysical profile with other types of antepartum fetal assessment. The use of the biophysical profile did not demonstrate better perinatal outcomes when compared with other forms of antepartum assessment. However, in view of the small numbers in this analysis, definitive conclusions concerning the usefulness of the biophysical profile cannot be made.[12]

Table 11.1 Components of the 30 minute Biophysical Profile Score

Component	Definition
Fetal movements (*)	≥ 3 body or limb movements
Fetal tone (*)	One episode of active extension and flexion of the limbs; opening and closing of hand
Fetal breathing movements (*)	≥ 1 episode of ≥ 30 seconds in 30 minutes. Hiccoughs are considered breathing activity
Amniotic fluid volume (*)	A single 2 cm × 2 cm pocket of fluid with no cord
CTG	2 accelerations > 15 beats per minute of at least 15 seconds duration

(*) Assessed by ultrasound examination

WHEN DOES FETAL ASSESSMENT FAIL?

All of the modalities described above are aimed at identifying gradual deterioration in fetal health to allow definitive management to be applied at a time when fetal benefit is likely. Despite much research into strategies designed to improve fetal wellbeing in utero, delivery remains the mainstay of management. Even with the most sophisticated fetal monitoring, acute events can occur that are unpredictable. Box 11.1 outlines the commonest acute events for which no fetal monitoring can be predictive.

Box 11.1 Maternal and fetal causes of stillbirth within 1 week of a normal fetal assessment

Maternal
- Placental abruption
- Diabetic ketoacidosis
- Sickle cell crisis
- Drug overdose
- Motor vehicle accident
- Acute maternal disease.

Fetal
- Fetomaternal haemorrhage
- Cord prolapse
- Ruptured membranes
- Ruptured vasa praevia
- Cord entanglement
- Acute twin-to-twin transfusion (only in monochorionic twins)
- Umbilical artery thrombosis.

It is important, therefore, that when these events are considered possibilities, a previously reassuring fetal assessment is not used to provide inappropriate reassurance and a full and urgent reassessment is made if considered necessary.

CONCLUSION

Screening for fetal wellbeing relies on the ability of the compromised fetus to make adaptations, which can be detected using a number of strategies. Whilst many of these strategies are in widespread use in clinical practice, few have been fully evaluated, especially in a population of healthy women. The lack of any one test with a high sensitivity or specificity for the identification of the compromised fetus means that there continue to be stillbirths and significant numbers of undiagnosed growth restricted babies born to women in the otherwise healthy population. The development of a good strategy to accurately identify the compromised fetus in this group remains one of the main challenges of antenatal care in this century. Whilst we await research in this area, we must encourage the efficient use of the tools we have and educate women regarding lifestyle modification (such as smoking reduction) and being vigilant for the movements of their baby. The myth that babies become less active as term approaches must be dispelled so that recognition of the first fetal adaptive response can be made appropriately.

Key Practice Points

- Antenatal care is the major screening tool used for assessment of fetal wellbeing in the low-risk pregnancy.
- Maternal risk can be used to identify women at increased risk of fetal compromise, and should be reassessed as pregnancy progresses, as new maternal conditions can develop.
- A reduction in fetal movements in the third trimester must always be fully investigated as it may be indicative of fetal compromise. At the very least a symphysis fundal height measurement should be plotted and a CTG performed.
- The SFH should be plotted at every routine visit in the third trimester when ultrasound is not being used to monitor fetal growth.
- Routine auscultation of the fetal heart is unecessary when fetal movement is felt. However, many mothers find it reassuring to hear the fetal heart, and in such cases a hand-held Doppler device is needed.
- Acute events can occur, even when regular fetal surveillance is being undertaken and prompt action is required when these are suspected.

References

1. NICE. Antenatal care: routine care for the healthy pregnant woman. London: National Institute for Clinical Excellence. RCOG Press; 2003.
2. Gardosi J, Mul T, Mongelli M, Fagan D. Analysis of birthweight and gestational age in antepartum stillbirths. British Journal of Obstetrics and Gynaecology 1998; 105(5):524–530.
3. Kean LH, Liu DTY. Antenatal care as a screening tool for the detection of small for gestational age babies. Journal of Obstetrics and Gynaecology 1995; 16(2):77–82.
4. Olesen AG, Svare JA. Decreased fetal movements: background, assessment and clinical management. Acta Obstet Gynecol Scand 2004; 83:818–826.
5. Ferrazzi E, Bozzo M, Rigano S, et al. Temporal sequence of abnormal Doppler changes in the peripheral and central circulatory systems of the severely growth-restricted fetus. Ultrasound in Obstetrics and Gynecology 2002; 19:140–146.
6. Manning FA, Snijders R, Harman CR, et al. Fetal biophysical profile score. VI Correlation with antepartum umbilical venous fetal pH. Am J Obstet Gynecol 1993; 169:755–763.
7. Grant A, Elbourne D, Valentin L, Alexander S. Routine formal fetal movement counting and risk of antepartum late death in normally formed singletons. Lancet 1989; 2:345–349.
8. Gardosi J, Francis A. Controlled trial of fundal height measurement plotted on customised antenatal growth charts. British Journal of Obstetrics and Gynaecology 1999; 106:309–317.
9. American College of Obstetricians and Gynecologists. Practice bulletin. Antepartum fetal surveillance. Clinical management guidelines for obstetricians–gynecologists. International Journal of Obstetrics and Gynecology 2000; 68:175–185.
10. Neilson JP, Alfirevic Z. Doppler ultrasound for fetal assessment in high risk pregnancies The Cochrane Database of Systematic Reviews. Issue 1; 2005.
11. Manning FA, Platt LD, Sipos L. Antepartum fetal evaluation: development of a fetal biophysical profile. Am J Obstet Gynecol 1980; 136:787–795.
12. Alfirevic Z, Neilson JP. Biophysical profile for fetal assessment in high risk pregnancies. Cochrane Pregnancy and Childbirth Group. Cochrane Database Systematic Reviews. Issue 4; 2000.

Section Four
Ongoing developments

12

Antenatal investigations for the future

Amanda Sullivan

INTRODUCTION

Antenatal investigations have always featured in midwifery texts. The ancient Greeks proposed that conception could be confirmed by keeping the woman's urine for 3 days and then straining it through a fine linen cloth. The presence of small living creatures in the urine confirmed conception. Today's midwives have a plethora of sophisticated technologies to provide information about a pregnancy. The first chapter of this book charted the history of antenatal technologies that are now integral to routine care. Later chapters described how to discuss, apply and interpret these technologies. This final chapter will outline key developments that are likely to impact on antenatal care and midwifery roles in the near future. Some new tests and

emerging technologies will also be discussed. To conclude, developments in genetics and ethical dilemmas associated with new technologies will be considered.

DEVELOPMENTS IN ANTENATAL SERVICES

Several key documents have recently been published that provide a basis for developments in antenatal services. These include the maternity and children's services' National Service Framework (NSF),[1] The National Institute for Clinical Excellence (NICE) guidelines for routine antenatal care[2] and the report on the confidential enquiries into maternal and child health (CEMACH).[3] Although these documents serve different remits and are produced by different advisory bodies, their recommendations include cross-cutting principles and themes that will greatly influence future service provision. Major principles include:

1. The need to target services to disadvantaged and vulnerable groups, in order to improve health outcomes
2. The requirement for standardised and equitable policies for antenatal screening and risk assessments
3. The importance of health promotion in pregnancy
4. Improvements in the quality and accessibility of information as an essential prerequisite to making informed choices about health and health care.

These principles are extremely important because they provide the backdrop for the delivery of antenatal care and investigations.

Principle 1: Services targeted to vulnerable groups

This aims to reduce inequalities in health. Currently, mortality and morbidity are highest in mothers and babies from low socio-economic and certain ethnic groups. In response, midwives have started to provide care from children's centres that are designed to be more accessible than traditional surgeries. In time, children's centres will be established in all localities and will enable a broad range of services to be offered under one roof. Emphasis is placed on promoting healthy lifestyles and access to health, education and welfare services. Antenatal visit schedules are also tailored to meet individual needs.

Hospital antenatal clinics are also being refined to focus on specialist care for fetal and maternal problems. Many antenatal investigations are now instigated and reported in primary care, with problematic results being followed up in the hospital setting. This places increased responsibility on clinical teams to communicate effectively and to develop integrated care pathways and referral mechanisms. It also means that midwives are acquiring new skills. These range from caring for vulnerable groups such as teenagers or refugees to caring for women with complex morbidities such as diabetes or HIV.

Approximately 25 consultant midwives have been appointed to public health roles across the UK. Their remit is to develop services for vulnerable groups, to work across traditional professional boundaries and to develop more integrated services within health communities. However, there are still many challenges for midwives to provide effective care for mothers with complex sets of social, medical and psychological needs. The notion of midwifery specialists is only just beginning to gain recognition within the profession.

Principle 2: A standardised approach to screening and risk assessment

This principle aims to ensure equitable access to screening programmes that comply with national standards. Some devastating consequences of errors in unregulated programmes were outlined in Chapter 2. Reference was also made to the fact that midwifery screening coordinating roles are emerging. National standards state that all Trusts should employ a designated antenatal screening coordinator, representing another expansion in midwifery roles. Key areas of responsibility are presented in Box 12.1.

Midwives' risk assessments are also crucial to the quality of antenatal care and pregnancy outcomes. CEMACH findings highlight the need for midwives to identify lifestyle and psychosocial factors that

---

Box 12.1 Key responsibilities of local antenatal screening coordinator roles

- To provide specialist care and advice for women throughout the screening process
- To act as a specialist resource for women and other health professionals
- To audit and monitor antenatal screening programme performance in line with National Screening Committee and Health Protection Agency audit criteria
- To assist with the implementation of new screening programmes
- To provide multiprofessional training
- To undertake continuing professional development in line with role requirements.

may impinge on outcomes. For instance, mothers who are victims of domestic violence have increased morbidity and mortality. Consequently, the maternity services are required to ensure that mothers are given the opportunity to disclose domestic violence safely and to obtain information about sources of help and support. This means that midwives routinely ask mothers about this potentially very sensitive topic. Another new area of midwifery practice is assessing risk of serious mental illness. Since suicide is now the leading cause of maternal death,[3] midwives are now required to assess the risk of serious mental illness and to ensure that all women with identifiable risk factors receive appropriate psychiatric assessment in pregnancy.

Principle 3: The importance of health promotion

This principle supports the need for midwives to develop their skills as public health practitioners. For instance, obese women (Body Mass Index >30 kg/m^2 in early pregnancy) are more likely to die in childbirth. They require full anaesthetic assessment and may need postpartum anticoagulant therapy.[3] Smoking cessation advice and nicotine replacement therapy are also increasingly available.

Principle 4: Information and choice to improve health

This final principle should be applied to every aspect of maternity care. For instance, information about how to contact local midwives should be available so that women with a positive pregnancy test can choose whether to access their GP or midwife from the outset. Options regarding antenatal care, birth and postnatal care should also be made explicit.

Women have access to an increasing amount of information through digital television, the internet and other media.[4] The model of shared decision making that was discussed in Chapter 2 will be increasingly translated into everyday practice. Partnership working with parents and pressures on consultation times will require women to 'prepare' for consultations through access to pre-consultation decision aids. This has already been introduced with some success in areas of cancer care. A recent MORI poll of attitudes to self-care[5] found that 32% of people often prepare a list of questions before a consultation. These were more likely to be from the more affluent social groups. There is clearly a long road ahead before true shared decision making becomes a widely accepted norm for healthcare consultations. Clinician and client roles are likely to change radically over the next few decades.[4] The possibility of web-based records owned by the client, who controls access to those records, is currently being debated.

NEW AND EMERGING TECHNOLOGIES

The previous section outlined key policy principles that will influence midwifery practice. Technological developments can also be very influential, particularly if they become part of mainstream services. Some new technologies, that may become part of routine care, are reviewed in this section.

Fetal imaging

Fetal anatomy scans at 18–20 weeks are already part of routine antenatal care. Chapter 8 described the structures that are examined and common abnormalities that are detected. Fetal imaging techniques continue to develop at a very fast pace. Some centres already utilise high-resolution ultrasound to offer fetal anatomy scanning towards the end of the first trimester. Ultrasound screening for fetal aneuploidy is also increasingly undertaken at this early stage. The nuchal translucency measurement, described in Chapter 7, has been incorporated into Down's syndrome screening programmes. Other first trimester markers are also under evaluation. These include the presence/absence of the fetal nasal bone. This may not be visualised until the second trimester in affected fetuses, as the nose may be shorter with delayed calcification. The broad face and impaired maxillary growth that is associated with Down's syndrome has also been demonstrated on first trimester ultrasound, by measuring the maxillary length.

A broad range of second trimester ultrasound markers for Down's syndrome are also under evaluation. These include umbilical cord thickness (this tends to be thicker in affected pregnancies) and fetal hand digits (these tend to be shorter).

Indeed, research into Down's syndrome screening has identified 40–50 potential new markers from either serum biochemistry or ultrasound. As such, screening for this condition is likely to alter radically within the next decade.

Conventionally, ultrasound images have been two-dimensional (2D) black and white images. Real-time ultrasound enables fetal movement and heart pulsations to be seen. This is an experience that many pregnant women expect and anticipate with great excitement. However, ultrasound technology has developed further to incorporate 3D and 4D imaging. In 2D scanning, the ultrasound image is made up of a series of thin slices and only one slice can be seen at a time. With 3D ultrasound, multiple images are taken and stored digitally on a computer. These images can be shaded to produce a life-like 3D picture. 4D imaging occurs when 3D pictures are shown in real time. This technology has been shown to help visualisation of abnormalities of the fetal surface, such as cleft lip and palate and spina bifida.

3D and 4D ultrasound have attracted a great deal of curiosity and media attention, stimulating debates about fetal development and upper gestational limits for termination of pregnancy. For instance, images can be interpreted as depicting complex fetal behaviour from an early developmental stage.[6] Findings include:

- 12 week fetuses stretching, kicking and leaping around the womb
- eyelids opening at 18 weeks (previously thought to remain fused until 26 weeks)
- scratching, smiling, crying, hiccupping and sucking from 26 weeks.

Despite these advances, ultrasound still has limitations. For instance, image quality is impaired when there is maternal obesity or oligohydramnios. Ultrafast fetal magnetic resonance imaging (MRI) can help greatly to improve visualisation of some structures. MRI scanning works by sending radio waves that are 10 000–30 000 times stronger than the magnetic field of the earth through the body. This forces cell nuclei into a different position. As the nuclei move back, they send out radio waves of their own that are then computerised to produce pictures. This is particularly useful when examining tissues that are surrounded by bone, such as the brain and spinal cord. Anomalies such as fetal cerebral ventriculomegaly or hydrocephalus can therefore be assessed using MRI. The evaluation of other abnormalities, such as diaphragmatic hernia and sacrococcygeal terratoma can also be enhanced.[7]

Fetal cells in maternal blood

Fetal DNA is present in the maternal circulation. Fetal red blood cells, mesenchymal stem cells, trophoblast and free fetal DNA have all been demonstrated in maternal blood. This discovery has prompted a great deal of research into techniques that could be used to diagnose genetic or chromosomal abnormalities without the need for invasive testing. Considerable progress has been made, such as fetal sexing and rhesus typing from maternal blood. However, there are still technical difficulties to overcome before invasive testing becomes obsolete. For instance, there is a paucity of fetal cells in maternal blood, so reliable identification and enrichment techniques are required. The size differential between maternal and fetal DNA molecules may prove to be helpful in this respect. Fetal RNA has also been isolated in maternal blood. This opens up further possibilities for the development of new non-invasive diagnostic techniques.

Fetal surgery and therapy

Advances in fetal medicine mean that in utero treatments for diagnosed abnormalities are continually being developed and refined. For instance, twin-to-twin transfusion syndrome was considered untreatable and was almost universally fatal until the last decade. Approximately 15% of monochorionic twin pregnancies have a haemodynamic imbalance, resulting in chronic interfetal transfusion.[8] Many centres now perform fortnightly ultrasound scans for monochorionic twin pregnancies from 14–26 weeks, in order to detect early signs of the syndrome and offer appropriate interventions. Typically, there is discordant growth. The large twin may develop polycythaemia and polyhydramnios, whilst the small twin may develop anaemia and oligohydramnios. Mortality has been substantially reduced by a number of treatments. These include amnioreduction to reduce the amniotic fluid index in the large sac and septostomy to allow liquor to pass freely between the two sacs. Laser ablation is also offered in a few tertiary centres, whereby blood vessels that are involved in the inter-twin transfusion are cauterised. These treatments have reduced mortality to 30–50%.[8]

Fetal therapy is also developing for a number of other abnormalities. For instance, in utero surgery for spina bifida aims to close the defect and protect the spinal cord from drainage. However, surgical techniques and effective tocolysis still need to be developed before this option is routinely considered. Surgical techniques to excise fetal tumours and treat lower urinary tract obstruction are also under evaluation.

NEW SCREENING PROGRAMMES

Screening programmes change to meet the needs of the population. The UK Sickle Cell and Thalassaemia Screening Programme has recently been expanded because haemoglobinopathies are now the most common single gene disorders in the UK. Haemoglobinopathy disorders arose within the malaria regions because carriers have immunological advantages and better survival following malaria infection. Cystic fibrosis used to be the most common single gene disorder in the UK, as carriers have immunological advantages against typhoid. Screening programmes have therefore changed in response to migratory population changes.

Service provision requires ongoing consideration. For instance, the National Screening Committee is considering whether to adopt routine screening for Group B Streptococcus (GBS) to prevent neonatal sepsis. Proponents of routine screening point to reduced neonatal sepsis and mortality rates in the USA, where routine screening is practised. However, approximately 25% of women carry GBS and it is difficult to predict the small number of babies for whom this would be a problem. Early onset bacteraemia in the UK is around 0.5 in 1000 live births and 10% of these babies die because of the infection.[9] This equates to a neonatal sepsis mortality rate of 1 in 20 000 live births.

Many centres selectively screen high-risk women, such as those with prolonged rupture of membranes. If all women shown to carry GBS in the third trimester received antibiotics, this could increase antimicrobial resistance and would be an unnecessary intervention in many normal births. There is also increasing evidence that perinatal antibiotics affect neonatal gut flora. This is potentially deleterious to regulation of the immune system and allergic sensitisation. Whilst it is clearly desirable to reduce neonatal sepsis, it may be that routine third trimester screening is not the most effective strategy when all consequences are taken into consideration.

DEVELOPMENTS IN GENETICS

Genetic screening is one of the fastest moving fields in medical science and also one of the most contentious. In 2001, the Department of Health announced that all pregnant women were to be offered screening for Down's syndrome, the most common form of learning difficulty in children.[10] Screening has reduced the Down's syndrome birth rate from 1 in 700 to 1 in 1000[11] and it is likely that new screening technologies will result in further reductions.

Fragile X syndrome is the second most common cause of learning difficulty. Affected males are generally unable to live independently, whilst females tend to be less severely affected. Several large Health Technology Assessments have been conducted to assess the feasibility of antenatal testing for carriers and affected individuals.[12] However, the testing process is complex. Fragile X is caused by a gene mutation on the X chromosome, whereby a gene sequence is repeated too many times. Normal alleles have less than 55 repeats of the sequence, whilst pre-mutations in unaffected individuals have 55–200 repeats. Full mutations have more than 200 repeats. Approximately half of all females with a full mutation have learning difficulties.[12] Furthermore, the risk of a pre-mutation becoming unstable and producing affected offspring varies between families. This means that prenatal screening for fragile X would present professionals and parents with a new set of dilemmas and decisions. The implementation of selective or universal screening is still a matter for debate.

Neonates are now screened for cystic fibrosis. It is also possible to screen couples for carrier status in the antenatal period. Indeed, parental DNA testing from saliva is already available commercially. However, it is not possible to screen for all mutations, so parents with negative carrier results still carry a residual risk. This can be difficult to comprehend and may lead to false reassurance. Methods for conducting antenatal screening have also been debated.[13]

Sequential testing, whereby only mothers shown to be carriers are offered partner testing, is one potential approach. However, this can cause unnecessary anxiety whilst waiting for a partner's results. An alternative approach is for both partners to submit a sample at the same time, but the second sample is only tested if carrier status is shown on the first. A positive result is only given if both partners are shown to be carriers. With this method, women must understand that they may still be at risk of an affected child with another partner. Consequently, there are complex issues to be considered before this genetic technology is brought into mainstream practice.

ETHICAL CONSEQUENCES OF ANTENATAL INVESTIGATIONS

Ethical debates are at the heart of decisions about whether genetic technologies should be introduced into mainstream practice. The National Screening Committee states that the aims of antenatal screening are to inform parents about the choices they face and to minimise the risk of maternal ill health or childhood handicap. However, Down's syndrome and fetal anomaly ultrasound screening give rise to concerns that there is an increasingly 'seek and destroy' approach to antenatal care. New genetic tests would add fuel to this debate. Certainly, antenatal screening can be regarded as ethically distinct from neonatal screening. Antenatal detection of abnormalities may result in termination of the pregnancy, whereas neonatal testing is currently restricted to conditions that benefit from early detection and treatment.

There is a very fine balance between seeking to promote choice and ameliorate suffering, versus the view that screening devalues the lives of disabled people in society. There are no simple answers, but the midwife's role is to offer available screening tests and to facilitate informed decisions

that are in line with the women's values. The Human Genetics Commission has been established to monitor and develop policies for the application of genetic technologies. This incorporates reproductive decision making. The Commission is also working with the National Screening Committee to consider the case for full genetic profiling of babies at birth.

Advances in genetics have been combined with reproductive medicine to enable pre-implantation genetic diagnosis (PGD). Following in vitro fertilisation, a blastomere is extracted from the embryo for diagnosis. Affected embryos are then destroyed and healthy embryos are replaced for implantation. This avoids the need for invasive prenatal testing and potential termination of an established pregnancy. However, PGD remains an expensive technique that may not result in delivery of a healthy baby.

Controversially, PGD is used in the USA for sex selection on the grounds of gender preference. Some restrictions are enforced, such as parents must be married, they must already have at least one child and must desire a child of the least represented sex of children in the family. This remains illegal in the UK,[14] although there are calls to make sex selection legal. An example of this is shown in Box 12.2. Other countries, such as India and China, have made termination of pregnancy on the grounds of fetal gender illegal, but the law has not been enforced.

> ### Box 12.2   Sex selection
>
> The Mastertons lost their youngest child, a 3 year-old daughter. They already had four sons and campaigned for the right to rebuild their family with a daughter. Louise Masterton had been sterilised and so could not use sperm sorting followed by artificial insemination (these techniques are currently unregulated in the UK). The Mastertons were unable to find a clinic in the UK that was willing to apply to the Human Fertilisation and Embryology Authority for a licence to perform PGD for sex selection. They eventually sought treatment in Italy and produced one male embryo. This was donated to an infertile couple.

CONCLUSION

Antenatal investigations are integral to antenatal care. The clinically competent midwife needs to understand when and how to instigate testing. The competent midwife must also interpret results and locate findings within the broader clinical picture. Abnormal results require follow-up by the medical team. Investigations are increasing in their sophistication and application. They should inform clinical judgements, not replace them. The way that midwives deliver antenatal care will undoubtedly change and will be influenced by government policies and new technologies. Antenatal investigations enable us to peek into hitherto uncharted territories and reveal parts of the mystery person in the womb. New therapies aim to influence the future of that mystery person. The ongoing dilemma for society and for individuals is how much we should peek, how much we should seek to change and at what cost.

Key Practice Points

- Antenatal care should be delivered in a way that meets the needs of vulnerable and disadvantaged groups.
- Pregnancy risk assessments should incorporate lifestyle and psychosocial factors that may affect pregnancy outcomes.
- The development of new investigations and therapies will continue to create new dilemmas and choices for professionals and parents alike.
- Midwives play a vital role in helping parents make decisions that may affect them for the rest of their lives.

References

1. Department of Health, Department for Education and Skills. National Service Framework for children, young people and maternity services. Part 3 (Standard 11). London: The Stationery Office; 2004.

2. National Institute for Clinical Excellence. Antenatal care: routine care for the healthy pregnant woman. London: NICE Care Guideline; 2003.

3. Lewis G, ed. CEMACH. Why mothers die 2000–2002. Report on the Confidential Enquiries into Maternal Deaths in the UK. London: RCOG Press; 2004.

4. Gray MA. The resourceful patient. 21st century healthcare. Web-based book and toolkit. Online. Available: www.resourcefulpatient.org/text 2003.

5. MORI. Attitudes to self-care. Baseline study. Research conducted for the Department of Health October 2004. In: Department of Health. Better information, better choices, better health. Putting information at the centre of health. London: Department of Health; 2004. Online. Available: www.dh.gov.uk/

6. Campbell S. Watch me grow. London: Caroll and Brown; 2004.

7. Kumar S, O'Brien A. Recent developments in fetal medicine. BMJ 2004; 328(7446):1002–1006.

8. Hecher K, Plath H, Bregenzer T, et al. Endoscopic laser surgery versus serial amniocentesis in the treatment of severe twin-twin transfusion syndrome. Am J Obstet Gynecol 1999; 180(3):717–724.

9. Health Technology Assessment. Antenatal screening for Group B Streptococcus colonisation. HTA Commissioning brief 05/05; 2005.

10. Department of Health. Boost for baby health—new screening programmes. Department of Health Press Release 2001/0208. Online. Available: www.dh.gov.uk/Publications And Statistics/Press Releases/Press Releases/Library/fs/en

11. National Down's Syndrome Cytogenetic Register (Wolfson Institute of Preventive Medicine). 2003 Annual Report. NDSCR; 2004. Online. Available: www.wolfson.qmul.ac.uk/ndscr/

12. Song F. Screening for fragile X syndrome: a literature review and modelling study. Health Technology Assessment Report 2003; 7(16). Online. Available: www.hta.nhsweb.nhs.uk/Project Data/3_project_record_published.asp?pjtld=1257

13. Marteau TM, Michie S, Miedzybrodzka ZH, et al. Incorrect recall of residual risk 3 years after carrier screening for cystic fibrosis: a comparison of two-step and couple screening. Am J Obstet Gynecol 1999; 181(1):165–169.

14. Parliamentary Office of Science and Technology. Sex selection. POSTnote 198. July 2003; Parliamentary Copyright. Online. Available: www.parliament.uk/parliamentary_offices/post/biology.cfm#2003

Index

References to non-textual information such as Boxes, Figures or Tables are in *italic* print